WONDERFUL *Little* SEX BOOK

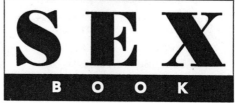

WILLIAM ASHOKA ROSS

conari press

To all my lovers,
mentors, guides, and students,
everywhere!

THE WONDERFUL LITTLE SEX BOOK
Copyright © 1987 & 1992 by William Ashoka Ross

ISBN: 0-943233-34-8

Printed in the United States of America on recycled paper

A portion of this book was previously published in *Sex: There's More To It Than You've Been Told*, published by Playful Wisdom Press.

Cover by Sharon Smith Design

Library of Congress Cataloging-in-Publication Data

Ross, William Ashoka, 1930-
      The wonderful little sex book / by William Ashoka Ross.
        p. cm.
      "A portion of this book was previously published in Sex:
there's more to it than you've been told."
      ISBN 0-943233-34-8 (pbk.) : $9.95
      1. Sex instruction. 2. Sex (Psychology) I. Title.
      HQ31.R8434 1992
      306.7'07—dc20   92-3948
                                    CIP

First edition

1 2 3 4 5 6 7 8 9 10

Introduction

*M*y Greetings to the Reader!
Good sex is fresh and alive and innocent, but you'd sure never know it from what you see and read!

Most books on sex are horrendous. They talk about sex as if it were plumbing. They act as though it's just a question of learning what knobs to turn, what valves to open. They reduce a human being into a machine. When someone who's a newcomer to sex comes across a book like that, it's like reading a manual on how to program your VCR. They *say* sex is beautiful, sex is natural, but reading such books you don't feel that—you perceive sex as very complicated acrobatics, a cocktail party without clothes.

This book is my attempt to set things right, to help you find the fresh, innocent aliveness that is your sexual birthright.

The world is full of judgment and condemnation. Especially when it comes to sex. In the realm of sex, practically *everything* is

1

judged. That's why so few people talk about it except with innuendo. And sarcasm. And lifted eyebrows. But they don't really talk about it.

When I was younger I wondered what all the hush-hush was about. Now I know everyone was always too embarrassed to talk freely. Of course, I was too, and I still often am—it is embarrassing to talk about sex. However, it's also very much worthwhile.

What I do in this book is talk to you about sex in a quiet way. I'm not trying to convince you of anything, I'm just talking to you about the way things look to me on the basis of my personal and professional life experiences. If you find contradictions in some of what I say, that doesn't mean I'm careless, it just means that sex is a very complex subject. For centuries we weren't supposed to talk about sex, and now that we can, we don't know how. We haven't been able as yet to develop an adequate language. In what follows I try to show a way.

Is there really anything new to say about sex? Yes, there is—lots! There's the whole *inner* dimension of sex—the personal dimension, the meaning of sex—and that is never talked about.

In many ways, we are only now coming out of the sexual dark ages. We finally have enough information to raise sex to a higher level. Until recently, sex was not studied at all. No one even mentioned it except in a bragging, macho, insinuating way. The original Kinsey Report was equivalent to the first sputnik, to man's first exploration of outer space; it was an exploration of sexual space. Since then, other researchers have made valuable contributions. But it is only now, thanks to our own Information Age of which talk-show hosts such as Oprah Winfrey, Sally Jessy Raphael, Phil Donahue, and Geraldo Rivera are the outstanding pioneers, that we are on the brink of changing sexual ideas and sexual practices in significant ways.

When I first thought about writing this book, I knew I wanted to write a little book, not a big book. I think there are already too many big books. I wanted to create a small, delightful, and useful book of encouragement that would provide many new insights into sex, inspire you to trust your sexuality, and help you experience greater sexual enjoyment. Sex is not simply "doing what comes naturally." Good sex requires awareness that is centered in the body. We lost touch with ourselves hundreds of years ago, and none of our instincts are intact. But now, through awareness, we can come back to ourselves. With growing awareness, we can move from bad sex to good sex, from low sex to high sex, from dark sex to radiant sex. Having been a curse, sex can become a blessing. Awareness can bring us from sexual hell to sexual heaven.

Virginia Satir says, "I believe that historians a thousand years from now will point to our time as the beginning of a new era in the development of humankind, the time when people began to live more comfortably with their humanity."

Living our sex life more comfortably is an important part of that journey.

William Ashoka Ross

SEX IS WONDERFUL.
Sex is *delight*.
Sex is about as close to God
as we can usually get!

*I*F YOU'VE EVER MADE LOVE ALL NIGHT and then gone to work in the morning, beaming like a fool at everyone and everything— cars, birds, people, fire hydrants—you probably remember how radiant the world was. Still exulting in those incredibly sweet and precious hours, most likely you had to restrain yourself from babbling to strangers, and you could hardly resist making a spectacle of yourself by dancing.

When you're aglow like that, you love the world. You're convinced that God bestowed sex on us to give us a foretaste of heaven.

*L*IFE ORIGINATES IN SEX.
Don't you think
that if this is God's way
of bringing life to the world,
there must be something godly about it?

But not everyone feels this way
and it's important to understand why.

*S*URPRISINGLY, OUR CULTURE IS BASI-
cally anti-sexual, and yet sex is everywhere. Advertising reeks of it: everywhere you
look, you see tight jeans and cleavage. A thousand loudspeakers are constantly blaring at you
"Sex! Sex!! Sex!!!" This is a daily pressure that
never lets up, not even for an instant. And if that
isn't enough, my dear friend, to drive you totally
wacko and completely around the bend, you're
either dead or remarkably healthy.

S EX HAS BECOME AN UGLY WORD.
Substitute *love play* for it and we'll all be a
lot closer to the feel and spirit of it.

Love play is sex lived with a different esprit,
a different zing, a new harmony.

Love play doesn't know anything
about forever.

When love play smiles,
skips,
and sparkles,
there is only
now.

*E*VERYBODY LOVES BABIES. THAT BE-ing so, isn't it amazing how many people are uneasy about the interaction that *creates* babies? We are, almost all of us, distinctly squeamish in regard to that very natural process.

How is it that we feel so at ease with babies and so decidedly ill-at-ease with the way they're made?

*B*ECAUSE SEX CAN BE ECSTASY, WE often think that the only way to arrive at ecstasy is through sex.

Yet what about the ecstasy of watching a sunset, tending a garden, writing poetry, or having a meaningful talk with a friend? All that is beautiful too. Still, for millions of us, sex is the most appealing and effortless way to ecstasy. Perhaps we have tasted something that those who haven't can learn from.

*T*HOUGHTS OF RIGHT AND WRONG don't go well with love play. That's one of the first lessons. Judgmental attitudes seem to diminish sexual enjoyment. But if you insist, go ahead—be right, have the last word, and condemn all you want to.

After all, it's your sex life!

*S*EX IS THE JOKER IN THE DECK.
It goes against our whole work ethic,
our achievement ethic.

Anybody can have it, regardless of merit.
That fact is very humiliating to the ego.

*S*EX IS NOT EASY TO TALK ABOUT. There are all kinds of taboos. There are words that are considered offensive. That's because sexual images have such a powerful emotional impact. So I wonder which words, what vocabulary, you will permit me to use. Whether you will feel more comfortable with latinized terms and clinical language than with ordinary words. And whether you avoid those people who use words that make you uncomfortable. And what that does to you—whether that makes you any happier.

*D*EVELOPING THE ABILITY TO LOOK
another person in the eyes—
not harshly or menacingly
but softly, in a wide-eyed way—
is tremendously effective in
enhancing one's capacity for love play.

By looking into each other's eyes, a deep exchange occurs, a mysterious osmosis. Try it—behold your lover up close, eye to eye, without holding your breath. While you do this, relax your face and body. You'll soon discover, if you haven't yet, why the eyes have been called windows to the soul.

*E*JACULATION ISN'T ORGASM. THERE'S a clear distinction, but being told about it may make some men angry. It's humiliating for them to think that they may never have experienced anything quite so rapturous.

Ejaculation is local, orgasm is total. Ejaculation is only a fragment, orgasm is the whole. In orgasm the usual you disappears, in ejaculation you remain present with your ego intact. The difference is enormous.

True orgasm comes from surrendering and melting and letting go and really opening up to your beloved. You do that by admitting that up to now you've been putting up a barrier.

*L*OVE IS AN ENERGY. IT IS NOT SOME-thing you can force. Love energy is a power you can become receptive to, because it is always there underneath the surface. Love energy is joyous, and joy is always linked to sexual feelings. What we call sex is but a small part of love energy.

Love energy also surges up in you when you smile at a stranger, comfort a kitten, or find the perfect gift for a friend. It is the warm, spontaneous, overflowing joy of a generous heart.

S EXUAL FEELINGS ARE VERY PERSISTENT because they are the natural flow of love energy in the body. So sex cannot be ignored, can not be repressed. We are abundant love; you can't not think about it. If you don't face your sexual feelings, they will torture you. If you try to forget about your sexual desires, you will become uncreative. Your every action will be stiff, awkward. It's these tender urgings that dispel your lethargy, electrify you with alertness, and bring you to life. Rejoice that you have them!

*R*EMEMBER THAT HAVING SEXUAL FEEL-ings does not have to lead to the *expression* of sexual feelings. And the expression of sexual feelings does not have to lead to sexual *activity*. Each stage can be enjoyed in and of and for itself—just as long as the emphasis is on joy. When you don't acknowledge your sexual feelings, when the emphasis is on obstinate denial, cold refusal, or furtive manipulation, something very ugly occurs and hatred is born.

*L*OVE AND TOUCH ARE INSEPARABLE. Similarly, self-love and self-touch are inseparable. Yet as children, when we touch ourselves in a way that feels particularly pleasurable, we're specifically told not to touch ourselves there. And any child with a bit of gumption will do it anyway because it's a natural response; we almost all do it. And when parents ask about it, we of course say no, we didn't, because we've been told we shouldn't. That's how we start lying about our sexuality; and once we start lying about our sexuality, we start lying about other things too.

Do you get the picture?

𝒴 OUR LITTLE SECRET—THAT YOU HAVE
something alive between your legs—is
everybody's little secret. Everybody is hiding this very commonplace little secret from everybody else.

Silly, isn't it?

*B*REATHING CAN HAVE A TREMENDOUS effect on sex. The deeper the breathing, the more complete the sexual experience. That's why some people say that relaxed and gentle breathing is the gateway to sexual ease. In fact, breathing can by itself lead to ecstasy. That's because ecstasy would be our natural state if our breathing weren't so shallow. Our present energy is actually only a fraction of what it could be. Take a few deep breaths and you'll soon see.

*S*OMETIMES DURING SEX A PERSON BE-gins to shake, to shiver, to tremble. If you're wise, you'll allow it! It is the body's way of releasing blocked energy. It shows that you're getting ready to open to your beloved. Before, you were afraid, even though you may not have known it. And fear was inhibiting your sexual enjoyment. Fear always curtails sexual enjoyment. Now, as you open to your lover, your fear is moving. If you allow your body to shiver and shake, the fear will soon be gone, and you will be far more vital.

*O*UR WHOLE CULTURE HAS BEEN ANTI-sexual for hundreds of years. It is anti-sexual because a person who is in touch with his sexual desires cannot easily be controlled. A woman who accepts her sexual feelings listens to herself and not to others. That's because our sexuality is so deep that we recognize it as a truth that goes beyond societal restrictions. Sexuality is a deep truth, and when you know the truth, you live the truth.

Some people think a person who does this is insane. They think that listening to the natural flow in your body instead of to the guardians of propriety must be an aberration. As a result, the fear of being condemned as either mad or bad keeps us repressed and timid.

*W*HAT STIMULATES THE SEXUAL APPE-
tite is sometimes puzzling. Sweet sex
grows out of approval and acceptance and harmony. Raging, violent, sadistic sex is a result of
hatred, indifference, and disharmony. So sex is
sometimes fueled by understanding and approval, and sometimes it is sparked by opposition and enmity.

There is, of course, an enormous difference
in the *kind* of sex that ensues.

$\mathscr{P}$EOPLE OFTEN AGREE TO HAVE SEX against their true inclinations. Sometimes that's because of the myth that sex "isn't a big deal." Don't kid yourself—sex is a big deal, and the fact that we can talk about it openly doesn't change that. Sex is a *very* big deal, and the people who have sex casually never realize that. They are devaluing their own currency, tarnishing something that could bring great joy into their lives. Sex is opening to a most intimate sharing, allowing someone into your inner temple. It's a little like bringing someone new into the bosom of your family for Christmas dinner.

So respect your own judgment and don't let yourself be conned. If you ever feel you don't want to, you *don't* want to—at least not now.

*H*ORNY IS A VERY GRAPHIC WORD. AND a very important one. In fact, there is no other word quite like it. It says something about a state of being, a condition many of us know. Isn't it interesting that so few of us were ready to acknowledge this condition until the word came along? That's because we don't talk about our sexuality; we are too afraid of being judged.

Here's another important word: *Intimacy*.

Because even if you have great sex and marvelous orgasms, what do you do for the other 23 hours and 15 minutes of each day? The one-word answer is *intimacy*, and my dictionary says it is a state marked by closeness, informal warmth, warm friendship, and personal familiarity.

Intimacy doesn't have to have anything whatsoever to do with taking your clothes off. Nor does it have anything to do with talking. When two people are calm inside and look with ease into each other's eyes, there is intimacy.

*T*HERE ARE BASICALLY TWO KINDS OF sex: exhilarating sex and "getting-rid-of" sex. "Getting-rid-of" sex is basically an endeavor to reduce tensions. That's all it does: it gets rid of tension, pure and simple. Sometimes that's necessary, because otherwise you get too charged up, but such sex isn't a high. You feel more relaxed afterwards, but it doesn't make you giggle. It doesn't quicken your step or make you want to skip. It doesn't slake your yearning.

Exhilarating sex brings delight, immense relief, and often tears of recognition and gratitude. The experience can be of profound awe, of having gone beyond gravity in some way.

*W*HAT IS THE DIFFERENCE BETWEEN "getting-rid-of" sex and exhilarating sex? The same difference as between friction and electricity. A lot of people think that orgasm is due to friction, but true orgasm isn't so much a result of friction as it is of energy. Orgasm is a function of love energy. We don't yet know very much about that kind of energy, but we do know that when it flows freely, it turns into ecstasy.

*E*CSTATIC ORGASM IS AN ELECTRIC, euphoric, tingling, sparkling experience; a moment suspended in time; a dark, pulsating sea of intense feeling; a quickening of the senses; a cataclysm; a gorgeous feeling of floating. Some report it "makes me feel weak and shaky and powerful all at the same time"; "cancels out all discontent"; "makes me hyper-sensitive all over"; "takes my breath away as it floods my body with dazzling sunshine." Some talk of an eternal now, of time standing still, of blinding flashes of light, of painful yet wonderful explosions of glowing warmth. Others experience being "completely in harmony with the universe" and "something from the beyond beckoning."

How can you explain an experience like that? Physiology isn't up to it. Neither is psychology. The more you try to comprehend, the more you are left with a sense of wonder.

*S*EX AND LAUGHTER GO TOGETHER. NO one knows why. Good sex just naturally brings up bubbling laughter in you. Suddenly you laugh at existence, even at yourself. And it isn't even because anything is particularly funny. You don't laugh the way you would if you were watching a sitcom on TV. You laugh because life seems so simple, so easy. Worries you had only an hour ago are totally gone. All that weight you were carrying has totally disappeared. Isn't it amazing? If you revealed this to your local psychiatrist, he might never believe you—he might even think you were mad! Something like this happening just isn't logical, and yet, it happens all the time.

*W*HAT CAN YOU DO WHEN YOUR swain's joystick has done its thing and he conks out, rolls over, and goes to sleep? There's not much you can do in that upsetting moment except snuggle up and put your arms around him. Of course, it's hard to do that when he's left you feeling like a disposable kleenex! But the next day, you can tell him that this simply won't do. You can explain that this kind of sex is a disservice to both of you, that you won't settle for it anymore. Blaming is a waste of time, but you can make clear to him how you want your lovemaking to be. Don't read him the riot act, but do read him some of the items from this book—that would be a very appropriate beginning!

*L*UST AND EROS ARE TOTALLY DIF-ferent. Lust focuses on a part of the body; eros means being moved by the whole person. Eros is passionately wanting to be with a person—intertwined, interacting. Eros isn't primarily concerned with sexual excitement; it is excitement regarding a *person*. Lust reduces the other to body parts. It is on a level with voyeurism. Even when the lusting person is with a flesh-and-blood partner, he or she remains stuck in a world of his or her own imaginings.

*I*N ECSTASY YOUR BOUNDARIES DISAP-
pear. Your heart opens out like a great sail
as your vital force mingles with that of your beloved. Your body no longer feels solid; you
become pulsating energy instead. There are
physicists who say that the universe is basically
not matter but conscious energy. Ecstasy is a
way of bathing yourself in that energy—a way
of being rejuvenated with God.

People sometimes ask: How do you define
ecstasy? The answer is that you don't. You can't.
Ecstasy is an experience that cannot be defined.
Next to being born, giving birth, and dying,
ecstasy is the most miraculous experience of all.

𝒴OU CAN PLAY ANOTHER PERSON'S body
the way you might play
a video game,
but you won't feel very good
afterwards.

*P*OWER SEX IS ANOTHER KIND OF SEX—
power in the sense of power over. Power sex focuses not so much on the actual sexual experience as on the effect that one's sexual behavior has on the other person. Giving in to someone's insistent demands for sex in order to placate that person is one example. Having sex in order to dominate or impose your will on someone is another. For example, a person who wants to feel powerful loves witnessing someone else orgasm, but this is ego gratification masquerading as sexual pleasure. Power sex really has very little to do with sexual pleasure.

*H*ELPING SOMEONE EXPERIENCE OR-gasm is a caring thing to do, but it may not be motivated by love or even enjoyment. It may just be a kind of indirect prostitution. Having sex because of what it does for another person alienates you from yourself and your own fulfillment. You may be doing it with a lot of love, but you've still got to be careful that you don't depersonalize yourself. There are many areas of life where being a Good Samaritan is perfectly appropriate, but sex isn't one of them. Unless, of course, you're a sex surrogate.

S OME OF MY PSYCHOTHERAPY CLIENTS have discovered that when they have been able to release anger, fear, and resentment in a therapeutic emotional catharsis, they are able to enjoy orgasm more deeply than ever before.

I remember a 54-year-old woman who screamed, stomped, and hollered until the building shook. Then she went home and had the best orgasm of her life.

Why does this work? Because a lot of our energy is devoted to bottling up emotions. When these emotions aren't squelched anymore, more of you is free to frolic. So do yourself a favor and scream all you want while you're driving your car. Vigorously beating up your bed is also a good idea.

*T*HERE ARE MOMENTS DURING SEX when complete stillness and silence pervade. No one does anything; no one says anything; no one moves. For a moment, both lovers are totally immersed in the stillness of the beyond. It is a little like those truly inspired moments when you're in church. Maybe that's why there are churches—to capture that moment of eternity.

*C*HEMISTRY, THEY SAY, IS WHAT ATtracts people to one another. That may be. But if, after the chemistry does its work, you don't rise to a higher level of consciousness, the chemistry will eventually turn into hatred. The passion will still be there, but the attraction will become malicious and revengeful. That's what soap operas are based on, and a lot of so-called great literature. That's what a lot of people still call love.

*G*OOD SEX DEPENDS LESS ON TECH-nique than on how appreciative you are. And to be really appreciative means that you are content with the present moment. You don't think about tomorrow, you don't think about the next moment; you're too involved with your feelings in this moment. Obviously, if you're straining for orgasm, you won't be very appreciative of this moment. You won't pay much attention to what is actually happening. But if you wait to feel appreciative *until* you come, you'll find that you'll have come and gone! Because, as you know, it can all happen in the twinkling of an eye.

*T*HERE IS NOTHING THAT IS DIRTY,
not even dirt.

If anything is dirty,
it is your own mind.

*H*ERE IS A STORY WORTH THINKING about. A man went to a professionally licensed masseuse for a massage. He was beginning to enjoy the massage thoroughly and relax in a very beautiful way. Then all of a sudden he remembered that when he relaxed deeply he would sometimes get an erection. So from that moment he was tense and apprehensive. He could no longer enjoy the massage. He merely endured it. He knew he couldn't possibly allow himself to get an erection. That would have been far too embarrassing.

Has anything like this ever happened in *your* life?

*T*HERE ARE MANY MISLEADING BELIEFS about sex. Some men believe they have to give their woman an orgasm, and some women think so too. Some men think it's up to the woman to give *them* an orgasm, and some women accept that view. Some women are convinced that a man always wants to come. Some men are convinced that a woman will be unhappy unless she has a penis inside her. And all these beliefs can be wrong at least part of the time.

In case there is still some doubt, let me say it again:

You don't have to have an erection to enjoy sex. You don't have to have a penis inside you to be fulfilled.

*I*MPOTENCE AND FRIGIDITY ARE MES-sages, not calamities. They are messages from your deeper self. Your body is trying to tell you something.

Don't you think it might be a good idea, before you go rushing off in search of a cure, to figure out just what that message could be?

*I*F YOU WANT TO AVOID POISONING yourself with resentment, it's vitally important that you always do what *you* want to do. *If you want to give to others, give!* But if you'd rather receive, then giving may make you resentful. Regardless of how nice or loving or generous you would like to be, you can't escape from being true to yourself. If you make love when you don't feel like it, something, sooner or later, is going to go haywire.

*F*REELY AND ENTHUSIASTICALLY TELL-ing someone that you love them feels great. It's a heartwarming thing to do. But when the other person asks for love, expects it, and almost *demands* it, then saying "I love you" starts to feel like a chore. Even worse, it feels like a kind of lie.

Love, you see, doesn't do well with obligations. And sex doesn't lend itself to rules. They both follow laws of a very different kind.

A GREAT DEAL OF ATTENTION HAS BEEN paid to the sexual organs, but the "equipment," as it has been called, is not what sex is about. You can experience sexual pleasure in many different parts of the body, not only in the sexual organs. When you are sensitive enough, you can experience delight in parts of your body you never thought of. When you are really sensitive, you can experience orgasm even in your nostrils or your wrist! In fact, you can experience orgasm all over your body. Workshops that include sensitivity training will point you in that direction.

*F*OREPLAY CAN LAST FOR HOURS. IT can energize you more and more and then even more. And after an hour or two of foreplay, you can feel so contented that there's hardly a need for afterplay—or for anything else.

*I*T'S NOT ONLY MISS GLAMORPUSS OR Mr. Universe who have something to offer. When it comes to sex, the visual faculty is often the worst for determining what is inside a package. What you see is *not* necessarily what you get. To find out what a man or woman is like romantically, we need to develop a kind of radar, a sixth sense, a sense for energy, and not only to use our eyes. In other words, you can train your intuition. We're all intuitive, but since we pay so much attention to the packaging, we often don't realize just how intuitive we really are.

S EX IS THE QUICKEST WAY OF FINDING out what someone is really like. That's why some people find it so alarming.

The mood changes are staggering. Scholars turn into satyrs. Tight-lipped viragos mutate into wanton sluts. Paratroopers are revealed as wimps.

You never know what you'll get—the other face of the medallion is always so different from what's on public view. The well-tailored lawyer turns into a monster of depravity. That prim and proper secretary becomes a screaming meemie. The contentious congressman, always combative, suddenly couldn't care less. Miss Hyperactive, mission accomplished, sinks into abundant sleep. That is one of the charms of sex—seeing people when their masks are off. Some say the contrast alone is worth the price of admission. You may not want to play, but you can't deny it's one of the best . . . well, maybe not *best*, but certainly one of the most intriguing, games in town. Everyone seems to want a ringside seat.

*O*NE MISCONCEPTION HAS BEEN THAT sex requires intercourse and vigorous movement. In fact, it doesn't. Tantra, a concept that is widely misunderstood, can be practiced even without intercourse. The connection can be through the eyes and the pores of the skin. Instead of peaking in a crescendo, the energy goes on reverberating inside the couple for a considerable time. There is very little movement but there is a slow glow, increasing, pulsating, building up, intensifying. There isn't the kind of abrupt orgasm that most of us are familiar with, and the experience can go on for hours. People who practice this discipline, the key to which is relaxation, sometimes have truly amazing out-of-body experiences. You too will probably discover them shortly.

A PERSON IS AN ENERGY SYSTEM. SO THE question is whether your circuits are functioning, whether your wiring is all hooked up. Have you ever seen what a logic board in a computer looks like? All those wires? That's how it is with sex: the external organs don't have anything to do with it. It doesn't much matter what size or shape they are; they are simply conductors.

And as soon as sex is seen as energy, the question arises of how many circuits there are, because people who have studied sex say there are many circuits and not only the genital circuit. There are *many* circuits, and much of the joy of lovemaking is in discovering them. You can't do that if what you settle for is a quickie. Discovering all these circuits takes time. It also takes a loving disposition. When you enjoy your love play and your partner, that's when new experiences open up for you. If you're disgruntled with what you've got, chances are you won't get very much more.

*A*RE YOU READY FOR MEANINGFUL, heart-moving contact? Then decide that together with your beloved, you're going to create a fun little space capsule of love energy as often as you can. How do you do that? You warmly hold your partner's hands, look steadily into his or her eyes—and smile! The smile is what does it. There are all kinds of smiles, and you can try out all of them. Stay together like this for a few minutes; continue looking, go on holding hands, and keep smiling. Creating this endearing little island of love energy from time to time will reconnect you with your soul mate in a very warm and positive way.

A WELL-KNOWN PSYCHIATRIST ONCE declared that if everyone
became capable of orgasm,
the world would soon be so loving
that both war and most mental illness
would quickly disappear.

That's because sex can be so satisfying that it actually transforms you. The richness of that satisfaction leads you to touch base with a deep truth in yourself, a truth you may have forgotten. When we are satisfied we are at peace with the world, and when we are dissatisfied we are at war with everyone, most of all ourselves.

*Y*OU CANNOT "HAVE" SEX. YOU CANnot manage it. It cannot be reduced to mechanics. You cannot master it. If you really move into sex, you disappear. And *only* if you surrender to sex, if you give up all attempts to take charge of it, will you experience what sex is really all about. Then your bed becomes an altar on which you happily sacrifice yourself with not a moment's concern about your purse. Then tears merge into laughter, up becomes down, poverty turns into wealth, his becomes hers, and all sins are forgiven. You can't fathom where you end and where your dear friend begins—and what's more, you don't even care!

*W*HY DO YOU THINK IT IS
that persons who are interested in sex
are so often dismissed
as reprehensible?

*W*HEN THE FIRST KINSEY REPORT CAME out a generation ago, it revealed that just about everyone was secretly much more sexual than had been anticipated. Until Kinsey, many people suffered horrendous guilt—they assumed they were terribly depraved, when actually they were more or less like everyone else. So these findings were very freeing to millions. And yet there were many people who thought Kinsey should be imprisoned. Why are such liberators always hounded? Because the book burners have always been scared spitless of their own sexuality.

*M*ANY OF US KNOW CERTAIN THINGS about sex from experience. We know that the more you have sex, the more you want to have sex. We also know that there's a kind of law of diminishing returns. The more frequently you do it, the less delight you experience and the more the champagne goes flat. You may still feel great and vigorous and vital, but the experience is closer to athletics, to what you feel after a good workout in a gym, rather than being like the ecstasy you experienced originally. Sex has become familiar. And if you go on like that, the day may come when it's a little like brushing your teeth or some other daily function.

*T*HE FEAR OF MOVING DEEPLY INTO sex, the fear of going insane, and the fear of death are linked. They all have to do with fear of losing control. Yet only when you discover that it's okay to lose control, that you'll *survive*, and that you'll enjoy life more than ever before, will you experience how truly magnificent life can be.

*I*N SEX AS IN MOST OTHER ACTIVITIES, enjoyment seems to breed enjoyment. I don't make up these rules and I don't understand their arithmetic, but from my observations it seems to ring true: enjoyment breeds enjoyment. This fits in with what Yehoshua (who is known to us historically as Jesus) said: *To them who have, much will be given.*

Sexual enjoyment isn't for people who hold grudges. If you hold a grudge against one person, there will be grudgingness inside you. That is known as malice and it will contaminate your love life.

*S*EX IS A JOYOUS EXPRESSION, BUT MOST sex manuals that talk about "the joy of sex," appeal to the calculating mind, to seriousness rather than to jubilation. Joy doesn't care whether it expresses itself sexually or not. The joyless person focuses primarily on sex because in sex he at least feels something! The joyless person can't bear knowing that he doesn't feel anything (or only very little). To a joyless person, even a twinge of sensation, a localized fibrillation of the senses, is better than not feeling anything at all.

*M*ANY PEOPLE WHO WANT RELATION-ships hope to find peace and harmony. But a relationship is also a learning experience, a war of attrition between egos, and sometimes that means friction and struggle. And sex is an instant barometer of that struggle. The struggle isn't only about needs—his needs against her needs; the struggle is also a conflict between higher and lower levels of love and awareness. That's why it's always good to ask yourself: What do I need to learn from this relationship?— and to develop some useful hypotheses.

*W*HAT MAKES A WOMAN THINK SHE'S frigid? Often it's her husband who tells her so.

Convinced that it's a man's duty to make his partner come, the head of the house's ego won't allow him to just go to sleep. So he tries to make his wife come. But frequently he's impatient about it. He focuses on her clitoris as though he were scrubbing a pot. When after a while of this she still doesn't come, he finally gives up. Tired, wanting to get a good night's sleep, he excuses himself and says: "I think you're frigid." So for a long time she *thinks* of herself as frigid . . . until she finds a beautiful lover who really cares. In a similar kind of way, a man will begin to think of himself as impotent. But sometimes, people never do find a sensitive lover. Then they never realize that there is nothing wrong with them.

P.S. The kind of "lover" who needs to be found may be none other than your very own spouse. Just a change of outlook sometimes works miracles.

S TIMULATING SOMEBODY'S NERVE END-
ings can become a boring job when it
doesn't come naturally. What's even more frus-
trating, it usually doesn't have the desired
results.

*T*HERE ARE NO APHRODISIACS. IT IS ALL nonsense. Diet can help; a healthy diet will result in more sexual energy, assuming, of course, that all other things are equal. But aside from that, the only aphrodisiac I know of that works is caring. When someone is interested in you in a caring and sensitive way, sex wakes up. A lot of things can turn somebody on now and then for an hour or two, but caring is the only thing that will *keep* someone turned on.

*W*HEN WE WERE VERY YOUNG, THERE was always something that made us feel better. It fixed feeling bad. So whenever life is rotten, we turn to our favorite fix—sex, food, or fantasy. Because the motivation is negative (not feeling bad), that of course downgrades sex. Then, with galloping speed, the fix becomes a roaring addiction.

Whenever your pride is wounded by some failure, your inner critic instantly whispers it's because you're *bad*. You grew up trying to prove you were good, all the while battling your suspicion that you really were incorrigible. So when the protective walls of your ego collapse and that anguish of utter dejection floods you, you turn to your fix.

That's why it's so very important to feel good about yourself. And you'll only be able to do that when you make peace with your inner critic. That's an art, of course, but as soon as you master it, no fix of any kind will be needed. You'll just enjoy.

*W*HEN ONE SHIFTS FROM EXCITEMENT sex to relaxation sex, there is a turning point. You feel the excitement of sex, but what you feel even more is a relaxed confidence—like going to visit a dear old friend. When we say yes to sexual relaxation, we are getting ready to melt.

Relaxation works wonders. The more relaxed you are about sex, the more at ease you will be with others. Then you will see someone, look deeply into his or her eyes and you will both *know*, even though you may never do anything about it. When there is total acceptance in the eyes, that is already sex, and more is sometimes unnecessary. That deep communion is often enough. Having shared that moment of intimacy, you are already lovers. And after that you will see every person you meet a little differently.

*D*O YOU REMEMBER THE TIME YOU HAD that perfect orgasm? The one you and your partner still reminisce about? The golden screw? Everyone who's ever had it always wants to reexperience it. And when we can't, we feel frustrated because none of our efforts work—and we of course feel they *should* work!

Some people think that's why it doesn't happen anymore—because we're trying to repeat, to copy, to imitate. If, instead of trying to recapture the past, we could be open to the brand new, to *all* the newness and freshness and awe that life has to offer, who knows what wonderful experiences might come our way?

*T*HERE'S AN EXPRESSION THAT SAYS, "It takes two to tango." You can't tango when you're not really in the mood; the most you can do is fake it. Sex is a kind of tango. You can go through the motions, but if in that moment you'd really rather not, it will lead to resentment and discontent somewhere along the line. If you want your love play to be as alive as it can be, if you want your beloved to truly love you, then *never* insist that your lover do something he or she isn't really inclined to do.

L YING DOWN WITH SOMEONE YOU LIKE and breathing in unison—inhaling at the same time, exhaling at the same time, in the same relaxed rhythm—will soon envelop you in a pulsating energy field together. Can everyone develop the sensitivity for that? Yes, everyone can. All it requires is willingness and, of course, time and a little patience. Even if it takes a while, it's well worth waiting for.

Try this: Embrace your partner for at least ten minutes. If sexual feelings arise, acknowledge them but don't act on them; just allow yourself to feel them. Breathe easily, deeply, effortlessly. Silently continue to hold your companion in an embrace of warm togetherness. Do this for about 20 minutes. At the end, affectionately thank this precious friend. It's a good idea to talk about what the experience meant to both of you.

*S*EX AS PURE ATHLETICS IS AN IMPOSSI-bility, but many think that they are getting a free ride. Persist in having athletic sex and eventually you will come to hate either yourself or the other person for everything that you're missing. That's as sure as shootin', but sometimes it takes years to find out. You'll have some kicks, of course, but your focus on impersonal sex will crowd everything that's worthwhile out of your life.

*T*HE WISE DON'T GRASP FOR THE FINAL climax. They know that the grasping approach short-circuits the delights of sex and limits its possibilities. They prolong the act in order to arrive at sex's deepest fountain. That magic fountain flows only when there is an absence of purpose and hurry.

Complete avoidance of discharge, on the other hand, kills spontaneity. Why set a limit to what may happen? A fixed goal inevitably rules out a whole host of unknown possibilities. This is as true for the goal of coming as for the goal of not coming. Remaining open to the flow, to whatever comes, neither straining nor restraining, would seem to be the most rewarding attitude of all.

*W*HEN I GIVE MY TALKS ON SEX, I often see people taking notes. And I regret that. I would like them to become more subjective because that is what is necessary for good sex. Science is objective and sex is primarily subjective. By continuing to take notes, aren't they conveying that they don't yet feel ready to move into the subjective? Clinging to objectivity is a way of being unable to let go.

In other words, sex can scramble your brains. At least the so-called reasonable part of your brain. And although that is sometimes scary, it is also a surprisingly good thing.

*T*HE FRENCH CALL ORGASM *LA PETITE mort,* the little death. That's because in orgasm there can be terror and dread and trembling as well as joy and delight. Sometimes the feelings during climax are so intense that you feel you're actually dying. Do delight and dread both have to be inherent in sex? Yes, they do, because sex is at the point where we are raw, where we enter into the holy and the mysterious. And having experienced that, having known that time when our personality was out of action and of no avail, we die in another way as well: we die to all in life that is not true, and to all old loyalties that are revealed as devoid of real meaning.

*T*O THINK THAT SEX IS MERELY PHYSI-cal and physiological is to miss the point. Sex is neither carnal nor spiritual; it is a meeting of the two. In the moment of greatest fulfillment, the other is viewed with an adoration usually reserved for God—because in that moment, the other has become an expression of God.

S EXUALITY AND SPIRITUALITY GO TO-
gether. Sexuality leads us to others, and
spirituality leads us to ourselves, to our own
center. Without the playful lovingness of sex,
spirituality remains abstract, arid. Without the
surrender of spirituality, sex may turn out to be
nothing more than a kind of interpersonal masturbation. The people who are highly sexual are
often on their way toward becoming spiritual,
whether they know it or not. Many a saint was
once a sinner.

Genuinely spiritual people are frequently
graduates of the universities of sex. They're in an
erotic relationship with unseen forces, with
energies that are invisible to the naked eye. To
the spiritual person, the attraction to God is
experienced as sexual, but this time the focus of
the attraction is not in the genitals but in the
heart. The experience of the heart opening or of
the third eye opening is essentially *sexual*. That's
the way it feels. Loving God, loving an individual, loving sex—it is all the same energy.

*C*HOOSING TO LIVE LIFE SENSUOUSLY refreshes you and opens you to the ongoing mysteries of life. That's why sensuousness can be the beginning of spirituality. Sensuousness leads you from your restless, random obsessive thoughts back to your skin, to your flesh, to your senses which are your interface with the world.

And spirituality? Spirituality leads you to your center.

L OVE IS A SCHOOL, AND SEX IS A VERY important part of the curriculum. What do you learn in the school of love? You learn to be more loving. The ones who don't learn it leave the school behind—they flunk out, so to speak. Then they spout rationalizations and justifications to confirm their idea that there is no love in the world. And of course they talk coarsely about sex. And while they do this—lovers go on loving.

To graduate from the school of love, you'll have to give up a lot. You'll have to reexamine everything you've ever been taught about love and sex—all the tinselly half-truths which are worse than lies. So sift through them, cut away the pretty pink wrapping, and find out for yourself.

*W*HEN WE EXPERIENCE ORGASM, everything seems to stop. For a brief moment of suspended timelessness, we enter a state of immense tranquility that is similar to meditation. Some even say, though of course no one knows, that in ancient times this experience was considered so marvelous that people wondered if they could attain it without sex. You see, in those days people inevitably got pregnant when they had sex. So of course, they wondered if there was some way of reaching that marvelous high without risking pregnancy. The story goes that this is how mankind first discovered meditation. The one doesn't, of course, exclude the other!

*U*NWILLINGNESS TO MAKE SOUNDS DURing sex—to moan, to groan, to cry or to scream—is a surefire, foolproof way of reducing your sexual enjoyment potential.

Are you *sure* you're really all that concerned with what the neighbors will think?

*T*HERE WAS ONCE A WOMAN WHO DESperately wanted just one thing. Did she want to live in a palace? No. Or to marry Prince Charming? No.

The one thing she fervently wanted, and she had longed for it for years, was to go swimming. She wanted to go swimming with all her might. But she told herself: "I can't go swimming. I'm much too fat. I'd feel humiliated." And she never did. She put on more and more weight and she never did go swimming, not for the rest of her life.

There was another woman who weighed even more than the first woman, and she thought pretty much in the same way. But one day something changed inside her. She said to herself: "I don't care if I'm fat or not, I'm going to go swimming. I'm not going to deprive myself anymore." So she went swimming and she loved it. Soon she was no longer bothered by people looking at her. And from that day onward, she started to lose weight.

*W*HAT IS A SEX PERVERT?
Someone who was once told that sex is bad.

A sex pervert is someone who is convinced that sex is something *shameful*.

He thinks that way because that's what he was taught. He is obsessed with the idea that sex is ugly.

And that's why he does ugly things to innocent people.

*A*CCORDING TO RESEARCH, MOST OF us think that *other* people have better sex lives than we do. Apparently that's a very common assumption, so please allow me to set the record straight.

Most people are not living in sexual paradise. Most people are living in sexual *misery*. Their sex lives are *not* great. If people were truly satisfied, fulfilled, and at peace, what need would there be for so many jokes about sex, so many films about sex, so much sexually suggestive advertising, and so much pornography? It's because people assume that others enjoy sex more.

So don't feel bad about your sex life—and don't compare yourself to others! Experience teaches that sex improves the more you're able to appreciate what you've already got.

I MPOTENCE AND FRIGIDITY CAN MEAN a number of different things, but there is one fundamental message: *You are not paying enough attention to your own feelings!*

Maybe you're simply tired, or you feel misunderstood, or you're under a lot of pressure. Your body is very wise and can teach you a lot—provided, of course, that you listen.

If delayed sexual response is chronic, it may mean that you have other concerns that need spotlighting *before* you move into sex—grief, for example. An unconscious fear may be saying, Deal with me! Perhaps you need to assert yourself in some way. But it's up to you to decode the information your body is giving you. Experts can only come up with some educated guesses.

*T*HERE WAS ONCE A RESEARCHER WHO wanted to study the effects of orgasm. So he decided to experiment with rats. He hooked up an electrode to a rat. Then he taught that rat that it could give itself an orgasm any time it wanted to—just by pushing a button.

And do you know what happened? Rat after rat orgasmed itself to death! Which is probably what some people do too.

My point is that sex can be life-giving, but the way many people practice it, it is death-giving. It depletes the whole energy system, and when it does that, the immune system gets enervated as well. And then, as everyone knows, any bug can come along and do us in.

*F*EELING JOYOUS OR BEING INVOLVED in a creative project, we sometimes temporarily lose interest in sex. This isn't abstinence because we're not trying to abstain. Rather, our own inner fulfillment is leading us to shorter or longer periods of natural celibacy. Isn't it odd that some people actually worry when this happens?

The whole notion of celibacy is very interesting. Though some people want to be celibate, others dread it. And of the people who opt for celibacy, very few succeed. If celibacy is chosen, it isn't true celibacy, it is merely avoidance. It won't really work, which is why there are so many guilt-ridden priests—and this is true of all religions. Natural celibacy gradually grows in you when you're happy. You never feel you're giving anything up. When you're already blissful, why would sex tempt you?

*S*EX IS NOT A SERIOUS SUBJECT. IMPORtant yes, serious no. A person who has a healthy interest in sex is not a serious person. A person like that may be lighthearted, loving, caring, tender, dedicated, good natured, and playful, but not serious. Seriousness and good sex don't mix.

*P*EOPLE SOMETIMES ASK ABOUT NATU-ral and unnatural sex.

Well, here's my answer—and it's very simple.

Doing something you like to do is natural. Doing something you don't like to do is unnatural. And if you have to experiment once or twice to discover what you like and what you don't like, I would think of that as extremely natural.

Just so long as it doesn't injure anyone.

*A*RGUING AND SEX HAVE AN INVERSE relationship to each other. The more arguing, the less good sex. Fight if you need to. A good fight clears out a lot of muck and gets fresh energy moving, but for goodness' sake don't niggle.

Here's my suggestion: Scream, holler, stomp your feet, get mad, throw things if you feel the urge is irresistible—but don't harp or quibble. *Don't debate!* Nit-picking is one big turn-off.

*O*NCE THE PENIS ENTERS THE VAGINA, the tendency is to go to it; the man thrusts and thrusts as long as he can, and the woman shrieks "More, more," or some equivalent thereof. That is the way most people make love, and that's what most people think of when they think of making love; but it isn't making love, it is fucking.

Nothing is wrong with fucking, and nothing is wrong with the word, either. The only thing that is wrong is that people tend to think that fucking is the only way to have sex.

*S*EXUAL MAGNETISM HAS NOTHING TO do with being cool. Cool is just pretending. Sexual magnetism is the outer manifestation of your inner life. Mostly it's got to do with self-esteem. You can try to copy what that looks like, but it won't be very convincing. Copying a style can take you only so far. If you want something that will attract people to you, try genuinely raising your self-esteem. If you do, you'll soon discover that it's the secret charm that works wonders.

*S*EX IS SUPPOSED TO HAVE SOMETHING to do with love, but just as often it seems to be an expression of animosity. Maybe that's why we snicker at dirty jokes; it's really a kind of sneer. We *love* the idea that sex is something dirty. It makes us feel like little devils, and it would seem that we'd rather be devilish than angelic. And our devilishness often propels sex.

How did this animosity begin? Books have been written to explain it, but I think the answer lies in just one word: *duty*. We feel animosity toward anyone who imposes expectations on us; and if we even think someone is going to, we instantly feel suspicious and hostile. The day society expected us to be good was the day we began being bad.

T HERE WAS ONCE A GIRL WHO HAD A craving for shrimp and one day she decided that rather than eating shrimp now and then and here and there, she was going to eat shrimp all the time and as much as she wanted. And she did. *She ate shrimp in the morning, she ate shrimp for lunch, and she had ate shrimp for dinner.* She mixed it with other things, of course—she had shrimp in salads and shrimp fried in a batter—but the point is, she totally went into it. And that alone—the fact that she gave herself permission to do this—made her feel great!

And what do you think happened? Do you think she still eats shrimp all the time? Do you think she has become a *shrimpomaniac?* No, of course not. One day she got tired of shrimp. Shrimp no longer had any overpowering appeal to her. She had shrimped herself out! She still loves shrimp, but it no longer drives her wild. It is no longer an irresistible craving. It isn't constantly on her mind anymore.

O NCE UPON A TIME, INTELLECTUAl who like to philosophize a lot (as int lectuals usually do) came to the conclusion th free and easy sex would make people mo tranquil. That reasoning seemed sound, so th advocated free sex. Soon *Playboy* magazine a peared and people started hopping into one b after another as though they were playing mu cal chairs. It didn't, however, work out as pected; in fact, the whole experiment failed w rather disastrous results.

It seems that when all is said and done, th is something dehumanizing about one-ni stands and the anonymous contact of genita

When affection isn't part of sex, violence is b

*W*HAT DO YOU THINK IT IS ABOUT OR-
gasm that is so deep and so moving
and profound that those who are in its throes
will again and again involuntarily cry out "Oh
God!" and even "Oh my God!!" I've been as-
sured, by persons I know to be thoroughly reli-
able, that even atheists will sometimes do this.

I F YOU'RE GOING TO ENJOY YOUR FLIR-
tations with the opposite sex—or with the
same sex—one thing is absolutely essential: you
must be able to say no. Without the ability to
firmly say no, life becomes hell. Unless you can
say no, sex is a constant burden.

When you've learned to say no, the quality
of your yes changes. It becomes a real yes. Only
when you are fully able to say no will you
become able to say *Yes!* from your whole being.

You see, if there isn't a deep *Yes!* inside you,
then having sex with someone won't really give
you very much. It will be just local. It will be
puny in comparison with what it could be. If
there isn't a deep *Yes!*, you will be divided—and
how can you really enjoy sex when you are
divided? Sex requires your total involvement.

*I*T'S NOT ONLY A QUESTION OF FEELING good—it's a question of what feels good where and how. Something can feel delicious in your genitals and feel rotten in your heart. Something can twinkle your eyes and tickle a smile to your lips without turning you on sexually at all. Something that sends sexual ripples up your spine can choke in your throat or clog your forehead. Lecherous sex is quite literally disheartening—your heart sinks while your stomach is sucked inside out. What part of you is affected by the other person? *That* is the question. A buzz in the loins is very paltry, and when you succumb to it, you're settling for crumbs. Whenever you're tempted by dark, leaden sexual energy, ask yourself if this experience will make you feel lighter or heavier, lift you up or bring you down. A few firecrackers going off in the gonads, some razzle-dazzle percolating your blood, is nowhere near as good as feeling the whole sky open up for you.

*J*OHN WAS A MAN WHO WAS AFRAID OF sex. He didn't know he was afraid of sex, so he kept chasing women who wouldn't have sex with him. These women were very beautiful on the outside but they had a cold quality about them—they were ice maidens.

One day John got tired of all this. He turned away from the ice maidens and fell in love with a funny, rather chubby little woman named Ellie. Ellie cried a lot and she laughed a lot; in fact, love flowed out of that woman like water down Niagara Falls.

Ellie certainly wasn't an ice maiden. She cried and laughed over John, and nibbled his ear and tickled him and told him how much she loved him. And whatever he did or said, she moaned and giggled with delight.

Well! Will it surprise you to learn that our hero soon lost his fear of sex? That he soon rather enjoyed it? And that the people who had known him before started asking, "What has happened to you, John—have you been to Bermuda?"

*U*NTIL RECENTLY, NO COURSE ON LOVE was taught at any university. Sex was sometimes taught—rarely—but not love. Even to have suggested such a course would have resulted in ridicule. Love was simply not considered scientific, and still isn't. Sex at least was considered measurable, but love was obviously unmeasurable, and anything that cannot be quantified seems to have no place in a contemporary institution of higher learning.

To be concerned with love is thought to be a little childish. And yet, almost all the songs we listen to tell us it's love that makes the world go 'round. And the churches we go to every Sunday always refer to a man who was very concerned with love. If we don't make love our most important priority, can we really prevent this world of ours from continuing to deteriorate more and more?

O NCE THERE WAS A WOMAN NAMED Hildegard who was frustrated. The reason she felt frustrated was that she always pined after handsome men—men who were always too busy or who wouldn't give Hildegard an ounce of attention.

One day Hildegard said, "I will turn to ugly men!" And so her life was transformed. She found great ecstasy with ugly men.

After a while the men she thought of as ugly stopped being ugly. It was as though, like the frog in the fairy tale, they had turned into beautiful princes. Maybe they had never even been ugly! One man in particular became very beautiful. She called him Aloyisus, although his name was actually Freddy. She had a few quirks, you see. Anyway, she and Freddy (a.k.a. Aloyisus) fell in love, and they lived happily ever after.

A frog *can* turn into a prince. Ecstasy is alchemical: it can change ugliness into beauty. Such miracles occur every day.

*L*OVE IS THE MOST IMPORTANT WORD in the language and also the most ambiguous. You can love ice cream, you can love baseball, you can love your car or your doll, you can love a movie star whom you've never met, you can love the way someone makes you feel. When the Bible tells us to love God, it obviously has a different loving in mind.

Love can be caring, liking, sympathizing, dedication, concern, adoration, supportiveness, or devotion, but it can also be possessiveness, obsession, desire, greed, fascination, identification, infatuation, or lust.

When you really love, it touches your soul deeply. You might hate the other person for being so obstinate, so stupid, but you love him or her anyway. Maybe only when you are burned in some way and *still* love do you know what love can be.

*T*HERE WAS ONCE A MAN WHO WAS such a good lover that during the act of love he was always thinking up new strategies for bringing his partner to greater and greater peaks of pleasure.

Did she appreciate it? No. "What's the matter with you, Herbert," she muttered. "Why aren't you ever *present*??"

Herbert, you see, was so involved in his orgasmic calculations that he was rather absentminded. He was like those tourists who never actually see those magnificent sights— whether it's the Alps, the Taj Mahal, or the Leaning Tower of Pisa—because they're too busy looking through a lens and going click-click-click with their little cameras.

$\mathcal{A}$RE YOU READY TO TRY A DIFFERENT way of lovemaking? A very leisurely way? Without moving, lie quietly with your lover in a complete sexual embrace. The man's penis should remain in the vagina for as long as 20 to 30 minutes. That's possible because there will be no movement, no friction. Only if the man begins to lose his erection is activity indicated, and then only subtle movements—just enough for him to regain his erection.

After a while, begin to move, but only with very slow, very soft and gradual movements—no vigorous thrusting. As this goes on and on, sensations multiply and become almost unbearable in their intensity. Eventually, this becomes so intense that you feel you can hardly stand it. It is excruciating pleasure, and you wonder if you aren't going to die from the very intensity of this overflowing sweetness. And that's exactly what's happening—the old you is done for, and it's more glorious than anything you could ever have imagined.

T HOUGH UNREQUITED LOVE HAS BEEN sung by the poets, it is only superficially similar to real love. It really is lust. Lust is the insecurity of having the hots for someone. Because we can't admit that, we call it love. But it *isn't* love, and it's important to understand that.

Unrequited love makes you burn with feverish excitement. Real love fills you with tranquility and joy. Unrequited love makes you tremble; mutual love makes you smile. Unrequited love wears you down; reciprocal love makes you soar.

When mutual love arrives, you suddenly realize you've been watching black-and-white TV when you thought you were watching color. You discover the truth when mutual love arrives beaming like a rainbow and you feel yourself melting. From a state of almost constant agitation, you've been zoomed to an Everest of contentment. Which leaves you feeling tremendously grateful. Grace has entered your life.

*W*E ARE LIVING IN A HIGHLY SEXUAL-
ized society. Money is the visible currency, sex is the invisible currency. People trade
sex for power, contracts, information, employ-
ment, invitations, autographs, prizes, introduc-
tions, publicity, dowries, travel tickets, loans,
drugs, rent, and even peace and quiet.

Ulterior motives abound. Mata Hari was
sexual in order to extract information. Schemers
have sex in order to get you in their power.
Gossips engage in sex, not for its own sake, but
for the thrill of later talking about it to others.
Buccaneers have sex because it's adventurous,
and weeping willows use sex to medicate pain.
Nice guys give in because it's expected. Push-
overs dread being accused of teasing. This is the
jungle we live in. If you're not firm in your belief
that sex is too precious to barter for anything
except bliss, you can get very lost.

S IT FACING YOUR PARTNER AND RELAX. With your left palm facing up and your right palm facing down, allow your palms and your partner's to gently rest on one another. Looking into his or her eyes, softly say the words, "I am letting go." As you do this, move your joined hands slowly in unison, so that as your right hand moves forward, your left hand is moving backward and vice-versa. Your partner validates your affirmation by saying, "You are finally letting go."

Take your time with this. Again and again look into your partner's eyes and softly say "I am letting go," or "I am finally letting go." Breathe easily and effortlessly as you do this. When it feels right to you, allow your eyes to close and continue making these declarations. Do this for about 10-15 minutes.

*M*OST PEOPLE DON'T LIKE TO ADMIT they're obsessing about sex. But the truth is, more people are thinking about it than doing it. In fact, even while people are in the middle of having sex, they're still thinking about it, wondering if they're doing it right, wondering what to do next, wondering does he or she like it, and so on.

Strange, because it really is a much better experience when you stop thinking.

Of course, nobody can just stop. But you can watch your thoughts without either blaming or praising, and without feeling you have to do anything about your cerebrations. Your soul simply observes your mind, which after all is just a big computer. It's called meditation. Once you get the hang of it, you won't be so bothered by your thoughts anymore.

*T*HE MOST IMPORTANT ELEMENT IN SEX is hands. Not many people know that. Having sensitive hands will do more to make your lover appreciate you than anything else— unless, of course, you are a virtuoso with your equipment. Everyone is hungry for sensitive, caring, delicate touching. If you want to be a good lover, you really ought to investigate touching as much as possible. There are many different ways of touching, and you might be surprised by how much there is to learn. In my opinion, they should teach it in school.

*W*ITH YOUR FIRST SEXUAL EXPERIENCE you learn that sex is very relaxing. But to use sex in order to relax is inappropriate. There are better ways.

We all need a release, but using sex as a means to relaxation is like using delicate transistor tools to change a tire. It's better to first "release yourself" before sex—not sexually, but in some other way. For example, when you come home all tense and hassled, sit down and start laughing. Laugh until you're rolling on the floor! Just laugh and laugh, even if at first it's phony. Do it for half an hour and you'll be in a great mood. *Then* you'll be ready for sex!

T HERE ONCE WAS A MAN NAMED Charley who, before going to bed with a woman, learned to say, "I want it to be okay for me not to have an erection." Charley did this because otherwise he would feel too much pressure. The women were sometimes surprised, but usually they smiled and said, "Sure." And, feeling reassured, Charley was now able to relax more. There was no pressure, no hurry, no obligation. That brief request spared him weeks of agonizing. And knowing that he could make this request made it easier for him to approach women. He enjoyed simply being in bed with them, even if nothing happened. And, much to his surprise, Charley was able to have an erection more and more often, and without even thinking about it.

*A*T LEAST SEVENTY-FIVE PERCENT OF sex is obligatory—just doing what you think someone wants you to do. He thinks he has to be a stud; she thinks she has to pretend she loves it. People kiss because they think they ought to. Ask around and you'll find a lot of people don't even enjoy kissing. Everyone's at a masquerade ball.

*J*EALOUSY IS THE FLY IN THE OINTMENT, the bull in the china shop of love. And jealousy in its virulent form can exist only when your pleasure is greater than your love. When your love is greater than your pleasure, whatever jealousy arises is harmless.

Passion is beautiful. Passion makes your whole body alive, vital, throbbing. But passion isn't love. You've read newspapers about crimes of passion: "I love you" whispered so many times, and suddenly it all turns into hatred and loathing. ("If you don't love me back, I will destroy you one way or the other.")

Once love is full, total, jealousy disappears. You hardly even remember what it was like. But that can't be forced or willed. The most you can do is pray for it and prepare the ground.

*M*EN LIKE TO QUANTIFY THINGS, AND so they quantify in regard to sex. The average male likes to quantify how successful a lover he is by how many women he's seduced, how many times he was able to do it, how long he was able to maintain it, how soon he was able to do it again, and so on. This is typical of the male mind, though there are women who do this too.

But sex is about quality, not quantity. It's about the quality of your energy, the quality of your attention and interest.

A lot of women say, "What really turned me on was that he was really *with* me." And you don't have to be superstud to do that. Genuinely attentive interest has a lot to do with it.

*D*ESPITE ALL THE DOS AND DON'TS OF society, when you meet your magnetic other, you will know it. The Chinese say that when a man truly meets a woman, even without any physical contact, a special magnetic force called *tsing* is aroused in their being. It is comparable to a radio frequency; they are, in a sense, assigned a wavelength, and from that day they are tuned to the frequency on which the other is broadcasting.

Just a look is enough to set that in motion. A man is content, has no concerns; then one day a woman looks at him—and from that moment he thinks of her constantly. When he does, he uses a familiar phrase: "I've got her under my skin." During the Renaissance they used the word *perturbato*, disturbed. They thought the blood had been affected.

Someone, somewhere, has our number. Maybe this is how God taps us on the shoulder to remind us that we are not really alone in this bewildering universe.

*S*EX IS AN EXPERIENCE IN WHICH YOU need to let go, and that's often scary. To really let go you have to trust the person you're with.

And you have to trust nature, too. If you're having sexual problems, one reason may be that you're working too hard at it. Perhaps you're not allowing your own autonomic nervous system to take over. And it can't take over as long as you want to be in charge and doing, doing, doing.

So here's what you do: you sit back, relax, breathe, and let nature do the driving.

O NE SECRET OF GOOD SEX IS RELAXING into your being. Once you do, you can make friends with your sexual feelings in an entirely new way. The energy grows and grows until you experience yourself—and your partner—at the center of a vast ocean of contentment. Then if total orgasm comes, you experience overwhelming bliss; if it doesn't, you are already so contented that you feel no regret. This way of lovemaking has been called sex *from* fulfillment rather than sex *for* fulfillment. It is totally different from the kind of sex where you "do it" just because you feel the urge or you hope it can lead to a worthwhile relationship.

L OVING YOURSELF IS THE OPPOSITE OF being selfish. When you love yourself, you begin to love others. In fact, only when you love yourself can you begin to love others. When that extends to the physical, it becomes a pirouette that culminates in sex. Such sex is totally different from sex in the mind. Sex in the mind so separates you from others that it can even lead to rape.

Healthy sex is the result—the inevitable result—of valuing fun more than security, discovery more than certainty, wonder more than knowledge, gratitude more than anxiety, celebration more than thrift. If you feel grateful for whatever goodness there is in your life, and if you dismantle your mental barriers, healthy and satisfying sex will come to you in a very natural way.

*D*IVING STRAIGHT FOR YOUR LOVER'S genitals is the surest way of committing sexual mayhem. It is an inevitable turn-off. Yes, it works, in a way, for a while—but usually for not more than a few days or at the most weeks. Yes, you'll probably get in a few quickies. But it's much too direct. If you long for the bliss of wondrous nights and deep sexual fulfillment, you'll need to build up the energy in much more roundabout ways.

ZEL WAS A WOMAN OF GREAT EXUBER-
ance. She was unlike anybody else. She
filled a room the moment she walked into it, and
sometimes even before she walked into it. When
Zel made love, she *really* made love—she moaned,
she groaned, she scratched, she bit—she was a
phenomenon. The way she writhed, you would
have thought she was dying. She was a woman
of strong opinions, intense emotions, and violent mood swings. But there was one problem:
no one ever invited her to dinner. Her number
one lover, Cranston, said this was because of her
excessive enthusiasm. "You intimidate people,"
he said. So Zel did the best she could—she
squelched herself, zipped herself up, and only
spoke when she was spoken to. One day she
woke up as if from a dream and said, "This is a
form of suicide!" She decided that even if nobody ever invited her out again, she would
rather be just the way she was. She got rid of
Cranston, by the way, because it was he, damned
fool, who had put this ridiculous idea in her
head to begin with.

*I*F YOU ENJOY YOUR FOOD, YOU'LL LEARN to enjoy sex. If you gulp your food or eat yourself into oblivion, you won't. If you eat mostly in fast-food places and flush down hamburgers and fries with soda pop, your openness to the sensory spectrum will diminish. It's your choice! You can eat strawberries so that you get a full taste by slicing them, which is a sensory experience. Or you can simply swallow them whole, in which case all that happens is that you ingest some nutrition.

It's all a question of how open you are to sensations. How much *pleasure* do you allow yourself? When you take a shower, do you let yourself enjoy it? Or is it merely a means to an end? All of that carries over into sex. If you take that means-to-an-end approach, soon there won't be any end that really satisfies—and not much sex either that's worth anything.

*Y*OU CAN LEARN TO ENJOY YOUR SEN-suality in each and every moment. Right now, listening to music, let the music vibrate the pores of your skin. Washing dishes, let the suds bathe your hands. Walking the dog, learn to enjoy being pulled. Every day there are hundreds of things you can enjoy. You can enjoy the leisureliness of a stroll, or the sweat of jogging, or the tang of a breeze. Every moment can be an experience that lets you grow in sensuality. Right now you can feel this paper, this book, this space, the sounds around you, even your own breathing. Being open to all that and with all that will gradually turn you on to life more and more.

P ETE WANTED TO BE A BASEBALL STAR.
He was great in the outfield but he couldn't hit. Every time he was pitched a ball, he missed it by a mile.

His father got him a mentor. This man watched Pete play and said, "You're so anxious to hit the ball, and you're so afraid you won't, that you don't even see it clearly." He explained that Pete's eagerness was interfering with his vision.

"For the next thirty pitches," he said, "don't even try to hit the ball. Just look. Stand loose with your bat on your shoulder and just watch that ball go by." After a while of this he said, "Go on watching, but this time when you feel ready, let the bat swing around and hit that ball dead center. Don't you do it, though, and don't make any attempt to hit hard." Well, it worked! And Pete learned a lot from that. And it went way beyond baseball.

*D*ISHONESTY SEPARATES US FROM OTH- ers. That is the only thing that is wrong with dishonesty. It keeps us in separation. Undoing that and becoming honest again reunites you with others. You are then able to flow together because you are basically one. You're still in different bodies, though, and that's where the fun comes in.

Dishonesty separates us from others regardless of how minor the dishonesty is. "Slightly dishonest" is often an even more painful separation than thoroughly dishonest. You know when you are dishonest, and that knowledge will have a highly adverse effect on your relations with others, including your sex life.

To undo living in separation, simply say, "I am going to be honest." Then note all your inner resistance until no resistance is left. No confession is needed except to yourself!

*W*E ALL WANT PRAISE, AND SO WE often enter into sex in the hope of getting some appreciation. You say yes to something you may not really want in the hope of getting what you're *really* starved for.

The funny thing is that when someone really praises us, we go all gooey. We tend to shrug the praise off, especially if we lack self-esteem. Appreciation makes us burst into tears, and we rush off somewhere to be alone. Compliments makes us all thumbs, so it's easier to jump into bed with someone—it's not so embarrassing. Especially if we've learned to play the game.

A fulfilled person is very different: he or she loves praise, just so long as it isn't manipulative. Fulfilled people know when they want sex and they know when they want appreciation. They know the difference, and they're not ashamed of wanting either.

*I*F YOU EAT WHAT YOU LIKE YOU WILL enjoy life. But when you are constantly denying yourself the satisfaction of good food, you become pleasure-denying. Denying yourself is going against your nature, and in time you will feel an inner resentment about it. Your subconscious, of course, doesn't know that you are depriving yourself, your subconscious knows only that pleasure-starvation is taking place.

If you deny your taste buds in order to have a better figure, that will make you more attractive to the opposite sex, certainly—that's the upside. But the *downside* is that subconsciously you will have hidden resentments toward members of the other sex because they're the ones who did it to you—they are seen as the cause of your deprivation.

And hidden resentments, sooner or later, show.

A RELATIONSHIP IN WHICH ONE PERSON always takes the initiative is unbalanced. If a balanced relationship is to emerge, the passive and active roles sooner or later need to be reversed. Being forced to always be *yin* and never *yang*, or *yang* and never *yin*, becomes boring.

Remember also that there's a difference between taking the initiative and trying to run the whole show. If someone's not in the mood, you can plead "Pretty please?" and do handstands, but it will all be for nought.

Sex is about interaction, complicity, fusion, and its underlying fascination lies in letting the other be alive too. Otherwise, you might just as well use one of those rubber dolls. It's the unexpected surprises, the inspired new moves the other comes up with, that makes sex so luscious.

*T*HE MOST HEALING SEX IS WITH SOME- one who believes in us. Another's high regard is actually talent-enhancing and magical. Psychologists haven't studied this subject sufficiently, just as they don't seem to have paid much attention to how powerful embarrassment is.

Embarrassment contracts and inhibits us, while having someone who believes in us expands us, strengthens us, turns us into gold. It is, so to speak, alchemical.

Someone believing in us means that at least one person in this vast universe feels we are worthwhile, naturally creative, and inherently lovely—that there is something beautiful about us. And that outlook rehabilitates us, even if we know that the person who regards us in this way is foolish, moonstruck, or a little addlepated.

M ANY OF US PSYCHOLOGICALLY IM-
pose a kind of Southern California
straitjacket on ourselves. In Southern California
the weather is always blue skies and sun; no
storms, no rain, no snow—just sunshine. And
that's the way we become if we're not careful.
Monotonous! If someone asks us, "Don't you
rain occasionally?" we say, "No, of course not!"
We're even proud that we never rain. Or we say,
"Well, *occasionally* I rain," and having admitted
that, we decide there's something wrong with
us—we're rainy kinds of people.

When you're not afraid of rebuke or re-
proach, you're powerful. That results in a better
sex life. When you are afraid of those things,
you're powerless. Being defensive curtails your
power; it divides you. Being willing to tell the
truth about yourself always makes you more
powerful and more appealing. A sage once said,
"The key to warriorship is not being afraid of
who you are."

*D*EALING WITH REJECTION IS NEVER easy. One way of coping is to become more inviting. Instead of getting mad when someone says no, ask, "Could anything put you in the mood?" That's possibility thinking: "What would have to happen to ...?" It produces a confident, relaxed manner, and confidence is contagious.

But don't push too hard for a yes, because that will get someone's dander up, and then their brusk disapproval will inevitably lower your self-confidence. Often accepting a no graciously will enhance your relationship as well as your self-respect. And if you're generous in accepting a no today, who knows what will happen tomorrow? The longer you can keep the sexual energy crackling, the better your chances will be. So learn to live in uncertainty and enjoy the sizzle while you're waiting for the steak. Pressing too hard is counterproductive.

*Y*OUR FOCUS CAN BE ON SEXUAL PER-formance or sexual enjoyment. Performance relates to frequency, potency, duration—quantifiable characteristics. Enjoyment is an inner quality that cannot be measured.

Cinderella is an example. Cinderella sat in the ashes, cleaning the house while her sisters went to the ball. Cinderella wore rags while her sisters strutted in beautiful gowns. But Cinderella had a capacity for enjoyment that her sisters lacked. They were envious, competitive, ambitious, whereas she was able to enjoy very simple things even when there wasn't a ray of hope. She had a capacity for enjoyment because she was not competitive. She had a high E.Q., a high "Enjoyment Quotient." Which, when you think about it, we can all have.

See how fairy tales help us?

E NVYING OTHERS AND FOCUSING ON missed opportunities is a mental set that will destroy your peace, your joy, and any relationship you have. You will see missed sexual opportunities all day long and you'll be tortured by them. A woman in black stockings goes by tippety-tap on three-inch spikes and your happiness is gone. You see a handsome man in a gorgeous three-piece suit, someone with the cutest dimple, and you gnash your teeth that he's not yours. This kind of hankering can become a constant torment. A lifetime of this and you're glad when it's finally all over.

If you don't let go of the fish that got away, it will eat you.

S IT QUIETLY IN A RELAXED WAY. CLOSE your eyes. Visualize someone you feel close to and imagine that person in front of you. Actually *see* this person, then look softly into his or her eyes and say, "I know you really care." Then after a moment's pause, add: "And I really love you." It's better if you can say these words aloud, but if not, practice them silently. In between these statements that express your appreciation, imagine yourself giving something to your friend—a flower, for example—while beneficent beams of light flow out of you. Alternate this with images of receiving a gift and from your friend. Be sure to let yourself feel your own face and your breathing while you do this.

*J*ACK DEMPSEY WOULD GET SO NERV-
ous before a boxing match that he couldn't
shave himself. A quail hunter got so nervous that he usually missed. A golfer got so
stressed she couldn't improve her score. All this
was due to excessive eagerness. The solution is
to practice in a nonstressful situation. That's not
so hard to create.

The quail hunter went hunting with an empty
shotgun. Since the gun wasn't loaded he was
more relaxed. After his first six "shots," all jitter-
iness had left his body. The golfer sat in her
living room, visualizing her strokes. Dempsey
had somebody else shave him.

Do you get the picture? Do you really think
your sweetheart is so unreasonable that he or she
wouldn't be willing to cooperate in creating a
nonstressful situation?

*E*VEN SEX NEEDS SOME TIME OUT. That's why sex therapists often ask their clients to refrain from having sex for a certain period of time. Actually this is a way of helping people get deeper into sex. Just as a field needs to lie fallow for a while to regain its agricultural potential, so do we sometimes need to recoup our sexual potential. Think of it as regrouping. To do this, take a vacation from sex, a kind of siesta in which only non-sexual touching occurs. Do this for one to eight weeks. Developing your sensuality through nonsexual touching leads in a slow but steady way to a greater capacity for meaningful sex.

*T*HERE ARE TWO KINDS OF PEOPLE. There are those who want to spend the night and those who don't. The ones who don't often start pulling on their clothes as soon as it's over; you'd think they could hardly wait to hit the streets. As they leave they say, "I'll call you," which you know is a lie. And if they do fall asleep and wake up the next morning in your bed, what's the first thing they do? The nice ones scribble a brief note of thanks and tippee-toe out the door while you're still sleeping; the others just leave and you don't know if you'll ever see them again. Or want to.

Haven't most of us experienced this? It drains all the gladness out of your heart and you say "Never again!" Which means you're learning to value yourself. And so long as you go on learning, there's nothing, really, to be ashamed of. The only way our wisdom can ripen is with experience.

T ANDEM TOUCHING IS AN EXERCISE that is highly useful. It takes about an hour. Take turns touching each other so that while one lover is the receiver, the other lover is the donor. After half an hour or so, switch roles.

The receiver is always in charge and can say, "No, I don't want you to touch me like that; I want you to touch me like this"—more softly, more gently, whatever the case may be. Keep in mind that in the first week or two of this exercise, genitals and nipples should not be touched.

The key to tandem touching is to do it over a long period of time—several times a week for at least a month. All sorts of strange feelings will arise, but if you hang in there, it will be worthwhile. It's very important that you resist the temptation to have intercourse, because that would abort the gradual buildup of sensations that is possible with this exercise.

*T*HE BEST SEX COMES NOT FROM DOING but from *allowing*—allowing the sexual energy between you to move as it desires. The best sex is like surfing: you go with the current. It's not like driving a tractor, it's more like riding a surfboard. You can influence the outcome by swaying a little here and swaying a little there, but you can't force anything. If you don't love the tides--well, the tides are much stronger than you can ever be, and if you don't love them and respect them, surfing will very quickly become a nightmare.

*W*E EXCLUDE MANY SENSATIONS. WE say, "Don't touch me *there*." Touched in a certain place, we get squirmy and ticklish. But sometimes it is in precisely those areas where sexual energy is repressed and locked. A lot of touching in these areas could release some of the withheld sexual charge. The thighs, for example, are an area in which a lot of energy is held back, and so is the lower belly. Allowing yourself to be caressed in these areas (and asking your lover to caress you there) can help you unlock that repressed energy. When this happens, energy begins to flow in channels where it previously could not, and sexual potential rises in the body. Gradually, your whole being begins to pulsate with more and more energy.

I F YOU REALLY LOVED ME, YOU'D HAVE sex with me."

"If you really loved me, you wouldn't be in such a hurry to have sex with me."

"If you really loved me, you'd take me to Paris."

"If you really loved me, you'd write my book report for me."

This is using guilt and emotional blackmail to get what you want. It always backfires and is totally different from "Will you still love me if . . . ?" which is more concerned with reassurance and scouting out the territory, as in "Will you still love me if I make love with someone else?" Wanting to know where you stand is always healthy, and it's particularly important in determining the (usually unwritten) rules in a relationship. Otherwise, how are you both to know what's permissible and what isn't?

O UR ANGER AND OUR OWN CRITICAL feelings tend to pull us away from the person we want to be close to. To avoid this, we sometimes blind ourselves to what's going on and don't put two and two together. We relate to what we want to see, not to reality. But in an odd way, this keeps us even more distant. Only by accepting our critical feelings, taking a stand, and sticking up for ourselves do we get really close.

This kind of fighting can sometimes enhance love. With self-assertion and good honest fighting you get closer, you become more loving. You make love more often. And with some practice, fighting ceases to be something terrible. You get to a point where you can laugh about your fighting just as much as you can laugh about your lovemaking. Then it's just something you do that adds a little spice.

*C*OMMUNICATION IS NOT CRITICISM, and your life will be a lot easier if you don't mistake the one for the other. Let's suppose your lover says, "I don't like the way you touch me." You can regard that as criticism and feel hurt, or you can interpret that as communication. If you regard it as criticism, you'll cry, get angry, and withdraw. If you perceive it as communication, you'll say, "How can I touch you in a more satisfying way?" or simply, "Teach me."

Quite apart from how long it takes your mate to learn to touch you in a more pleasing way, just the fact that you accept what he or she said as communication rather than criticism will already bring you closer. The important thing to remember is that a message is not necessarily a putdown, even if at first it feels that way. If you behave as though it isn't, you'll disarm anyone who's trying to belittle you, and that will be doing both of you a great service.

*H*AVE YOU NOTICED HOW, RIGHT AFTER really good sex, you fall into a deep sleep that is exquisitely innocent and refreshing? And how when you wake up and you look at your beloved, everything is sunny and warm and glorious even though there may be a blizzard outside? And how full of promise life is in that precious moment? How *easy* everything seems? If you've ever experienced that, anchor yourself in the memory of that moment so that it's there for you whenever you feel down. And if you've never had that, realize that this rapturous world of supreme wonder does exist and that it may open for you tomorrow. In that enchanted moment you have no problems, no enemies, nothing to prove or achieve.

Gloria in excelsis!

A WOMAN IS A *PERSON*. A MAN IS A *person*. Every single individual on this planet is a *person*. So don't approach sex with the idea that men want such and such or that women want this and that. It may not be at all true of the man or woman you are with. Saying something like "Women like it when you" may be totally inappropriate. So is saying "Men always" Yes, members of the other sex may have hurt you, even oppressed you. But for your own sake, you need to relate to each and every lover and prospective lover as an individual.

*L*OUISE WAS A WOMAN WHO NEVER asked for what she wanted. By a curious coincidence, she married a man who was exactly the same. Both thought the other should be a mind reader. Unfortunately, neither had that ability. Over the years, they both got more and more cranky. Instead of asking for what they wanted, they complained. He fumed when she served chicken. "Why do you drive so fast when you know I'm scared?" she nagged. The truth was they both felt sexually deprived, but they couldn't say that.

If you never ask for what you want, you may never get what you need. Worse, your failure to make demands leads to a kind of chronic emotional neediness—you never explicitly request anything, but your manner is constantly demanding. And if that happens, it's likely that you'll whine and get snippy, and people will avoid you. Wouldn't you rather ask directly for what you want? After all, you might just get it.

S EX REALLY COMES INTO ITS OWN WHEN you're able to allow involuntary movements. Then your whole body takes off and things happen that you had never even imagined. Every athlete knows that the body is a vast storehouse of untapped capabilities, and this is one of them. If you allow spontaneous quivers and spasms, they will lead you to truly astonishing peak experiences.

To pave the way for that, try these exercises. Lie on your stomach with your knees bent, your lower legs straight up. Spread your legs a bit, breathe, and you will soon feel light tremors. Then lie on your back (knees up, feet apart, mouth slightly open, arms extended upward and to the sides) and welcome the whole sky. Soon your arms will begin to tremble, and if you then alternately raise your pelvis and thrust it down again, the trembling in your arms will spread to the rest of your body. All this will prepare you to allow involuntary movements more easily.

*O*UR EARLIEST EXPERIENCE OF SEX WAS giving ourselves pleasure and then being found out and punished for it. If we weren't punished, we were reprimanded or, at best, ridiculed. In some way we were given the clear message that what we were doing was either pathetic or disgusting or bad.

This is our common heritage. And I mean *everyone*. This is the root cause of all our attitudes toward sex.

Well, now that you've grown up, look at all this again. Ask yourself: what in heaven is wrong about a child wanting to enjoy a few pleasurable sensations in his or her own body? Why do we have to interfere?

I F YOU'RE INSECURE, CELEBRATE THE fact. Rejoice in your feeling of insecurity! Be glad you can admit it. For many reasons it's actually good to be insecure—it shows you're vulnerable. And if you're vulnerable, you can grow.

Vulnerable means feeling alive. And regardless of whatever sputtering objections your mind may raise, allowing your vulnerability to show by talking honestly about yourself with a trusted friend is the most enduring way of bonding with someone. The alternating of tears and laughter is what does it. You don't need to reveal all your secrets, but you do need to show that you care and how much you sometimes feel wounded.

*M*ANY WOMEN TRADE SEX FOR LOVE, hoping that this will work. Usually it doesn't, and every smart woman knows that it probably won't, but that's the dream: If I have sex with him, maybe he will love me. Most men, of course, are only too happy to encourage this dream. Why not? That's part of the old macho policy of getting as much as you can. Since men are hunters, they're often more interested in the chase than in love.

Anyway, that's the way the game is played, as most of us know and all of us find out.

So a woman often has only two choices. She can trade sex for love or she can refuse to trade sex for love. in which case, of course, she is usually called a tease. A clear lose-lose situation. The point is that when you adopt a trading mentality to obtain love, you're bound to lose. Love simply cannot be traded.

*A*LL HATERS ARE SEXUALLY FRUSTRATED. All those grumpy, hostile, negative, cranky, sarcastic, cantankerous people who love giving you a hard time: they are *all* sexually frustrated! Significantly, their frustration exists because of inner conflicts, and only very rarely because of outer circumstances. All the people who hate are deeply uneasy about their own sexuality. Someone who accepts his or her sexuality and is able to move deeply into sex doesn't hate; it is impossible.

But simply having lots of sex doesn't mean you accept your sexuality. Even having boatloads of sex will not free anyone of hating; the inner sexual conflicts must first be resolved. This means you must first perceive that instead of being something ugly or dirty, sex is really beautiful. Just *having* sex will not change anybody.

*I*F THERE ISN'T MUCH ENERGY ANYMORE between you and Mr. or Ms. Special, it may be because of resentments.

Here's the cure. It's called amnesia.

First of all, imagine you don't know your mate at all. Look at your beloved as though you had never seen him or her before. Pretend you are strangers. Wonder to yourself what her kiss would feel like, how he might approach you. Drop every idea that you know anything at all about him. Look at her and see a completely new person. Every time your mind tells you that you know what your chum is like, say to yourself, This is someone I don't know. Look on your lover as a mystery. The truth is we are *all* a mystery.

*U*LTIMATELY, THERE ARE ONLY TWO reasons to resist temptation: that you like your life the way it already is, and that you're extremely tired.

*W*AS IT AS GOOD AS THE LAST TIME?"
   "Was it as good as the first time?"
"Was it as good as it should have been?"
"Did it last long enough?"
"Did we do it often enough?"
"Who was better, me or her?"
"It wasn't the worst you ever had, was it?"
"You don't hate me now, do you?"

If these are questions you ask your lover, *stop immediately!* All these questions are either statistical or comparative. They all convert sexual art into computer science. If you persist in asking them, you'll be digging your own grave— and that of your relationship.

S EX IS THE ONE AREA IN LIFE WHERE EVeryone is judged in regard to just about everything. Too much, not enough, the wrong kind, the wrong way, the wrong time, the wrong occasion, too aggressive, not bold enough, too inhibited, too straight, too needy, too thin, too fat, too flaky, too old, too crazy, too promiscuous, too parsimonious, and finally the grandaddy of all sexual judgements, *perverted*. To a judge, everyone else is either undersexed or oversexed—usually (but not always) the latter—and only the judge is doing things right. What kind of playfulness do you think is possible when you're stuffed with such attitudes?

*D*O YOU FEEL FRUSTRATED, MR. Johnson?" asked the sex counselor.

"Yes," said the husband, "I sure do! Sometimes I realize five or six weeks have gone by without our doing anything, if you know what I mean."

"I think I understand, Mr. Johnson," said the counselor. "In other words, you get statistically frustrated. I see—but do you also get sexually frustrated?"

Sex is an expression of who you are. If you concern yourself with a statistical ideal ("Is three times a week normal?") you are not being who you are; you are trying to walk on stilts to fit your idea of normal.

A FAMOUS EXPERIMENT IN A MAJOR FAC-tory found that increasing the lighting improved work performance. So everybody said, *"Aha, we need better lighting!"* A logical conclusion but not the correct one, because the really interesting finding was that decreasing the lighting also improved performance. What made the difference was change itself. This experiment is known as the Hawthorne effect. I will let you draw your own conclusions about how it applies to sex.

*Y*OU HEAR A LOT OF PEOPLE SAY, "YOU can have it all." That's trendy new-age talk. But if you're conflicted about sex, longing for it yet scared or squeamish, then you're divided and not at peace, which means there's hardly a single "you" there. If you aren't at peace with your sexual desires, the only "you" will be a torn, fragmented, deeply tormented you, and that's no fun. What point would there be to having all the riches in the world when you're in that state?

So friends, before you start knocking yourself out to have "it" all, why don't you do something about having *you* all? You can do that by finding someone who will help you understand why you have these inner conflicts. The sooner you're rid of them, the better!

*Y*OU *SHOULD* FEEL A CERTAIN WAY? Why should you feel a certain way? Where was it ordained? Was it written in the stars? Who told you you were supposed to feel what you didn't feel? Who told you what you were supposed to feel? Who decreed it? Who laid it down that you should even care about the opinions of others?

How you feel is up to you. No one else has anything to say about it. And in a sense it isn't even up to you. *How you feel is simply how you feel.* That's it! And when you get that, when you fully appreciate and honor that, you will instantly be a stronger and far more fulfilled human being. Because even more important than what you feel is how you feel about what you feel. When you feel okay about what your feelings, *regardless* of what they are, your self-esteem is unassailable.

*D*URING HER MARRIAGE, NANCY HAD been a doormat. She tried to hold her husband Jim by saying, in effect, "Use me!" Which he did, of course. But that wasn't enough to calm Nancy's gnawing insecurity, and soon she was doing everything she could to get him to use her more and more and still more.

One day Jim couldn't take it any longer. Feeling devoured, he walked out on Nancy and never came back. She of course didn't understand why and became very depressed. Then one day when a man showed interest, Nancy's depression lifted dramatically. But this time she wasn't interested in being a doormat; this time she was going after revenge. The sex was only so-so, but Nancy had discovered that retaliation could cure depression, and she put that lesson to work with a vengeance. By the time the first anniversary of her divorce rolled around, the former doormat had gone through 37 men. I just wish I could say she enjoyed every minute of it.

$\mathcal{B}$ ECAUSE SOCIETY NEEDS PEOPLE WHO don't rock the boat, it imposes its rules and values on us as we grow up. And the only thing—the *only* thing—we possess to counteract this is our feelings. Only our feelings protect us from society's peer pressure. And at the core of our feelings is our sexuality. So this tiny voice inside you, which is your sexuality, is like a David standing up to Goliath.

That's why there is—and has been down through the ages—such a determined attempt to squelch sex and to confine it to reproduction. Hitler was very opposed to what he called "sexual decadence," and when he took power, he immediately jailed anyone who was in any way identified with sex. All repressive regimes have indignantly opposed sexual education and sexual celebration; they loathe the erotic. That's because they know sex is a spark that can ignite rebellion—or rather, that sex is synonymous with rebellion.

T HEY DON'T TELL YOU WHEN YOU GET married about the *"Not tonight, dear,"* game that you and your spouse may soon start playing.

It begins gently enough with "Dear, I'm really not in the mood." But it very quickly turns into the annoyed "Jack!" or the dishrag sigh of, "Well, if you need it *that* badly." Then it graduates to the disgusted "You sure have a knack," which is code for "You sure have a knack for picking the wrong moment." The next stage is the huffy "Don't you *understand* ...?" repertoire, as in "Don't you understand I'm also a mother?" Then it escalates to the patronizing "Can't you understand I have *work* to do?" The ultimate put-down is probably "For God's sake, Homer! Don't you *ever* think about anything else?"

Can you invent ways of saying no that don't squelch the other person? It really is well worth your efforts to find kinder ways of communicating what mood you're in.

*O*NE OF THE BIGGEST TURN-ONS IS having someone think you're witty; it ups the voltage instantly. "What really turns me on," I've heard a lot of women say, "is when a man sees I'm really very funny." Men feel exactly the same way. When someone understands your sense of humor, there's an instant fusion, because you know that they know. What do they know? They know your heart! They know you're intelligent, unique, and fun to be with. They dig you, in short, and you feel spectacular. I mean like royalty.

Try saying to someone: "You're really very funny," and you'll see a blush of pleasure light up his or her face. It's just such an incredible delight when someone finally *recognizes* us.

S EX TOUCHES US SO DEEPLY THAT IT can become highly addictive. It tends to create a intimate bond before we are sure we want one. The other person may or may not be right for us, but by having sex a bond begins to form that may continue for years. And if you don't get addicted, perhaps your date will. So if you don't want to be enmeshed with the wrong person for years, find out about this person—his dreams, her fears, his quirks, her values—*before* you have sex.

But people rarely do. We are often so hungry, so needy, so eager for even a morsel, that we rush into sex and find ourselves—sometimes for life—in a relationship we never wanted to be in.

*S*EX IS A MYSTERIOUS FORCE THAT SUDdenly makes intimates out of strangers. And, just as quickly, it turns intimates into deadly enemies. Hell has no fury like a woman scorned, goes the saying.

Cast-off lovers are particularly prone to violence. If you no longer want to make love with someone, be very careful. When you want to end it, your Casanova may not let you. If you even hint you want to terminate, a cold annihilating rage may arise in her, and suddenly, the pussycat has turned into a tiger. You then find yourself feeding the tiger so it won't snarl and bite. You say, "Nice tiger, nice, *nice.*" Many people have spent years feeding tigers, to no avail. You can feed the tiger as much as you want, the fact remains you still have a tiger by the tail. A fatal attraction. And until you finally get rid of the tiger, you'll be living in fear.

L OW SEX IS SOMETHING YOU DO *TO* THE other or take *from* the other. Low sex consists of using the other. Low sex comes from deprivation and expresses itself in exploitation, grabbing, sucking, and a determined effort to obtain what one was previously deprived of.

High sex is the joy of giving rather than using the other. High sex is the delight of seeing that you're turning someone on. High sex basks in warm appreciation and is constantly and astonishingly harmonious. High sex is about mutuality, laughter, being in sync, playing peekaboo, doing something together. Your joy is in the delight of sharing an amazing journey.

T HERE IS A RELATIONSHIP BETWEEN SEX and money. Basically it's a kind of reverse relationship: the more people repress sex, the more interested they are in money. And the more people are fulfilled in sex, the less interested they are in money.

In a society where sex is repressed, making and safeguarding money become terribly important activities. When you're sexually fulfilled, you feel good about everyone and you know there's enough to go around. When you're not, you can become a highly competitive workaholic, always afraid somebody will—you should excuse the expression—screw you.

*K*ISSING CAN BE WONDERFUL OR AW-ful, heavenly or horrendous. Unfortunately, most people have never learned to kiss; they kiss in very boring ways. The timid ones slop their lips together, the more daring ones exchange saliva. The really aggressive ones act like they're drilling for oil; they hardly allow you to breathe.

A good kiss should be as soft and tender as the petals of a rose. A good kiss should be like the touch of a butterfly's wing. Sometimes (and it depends on circumstance) there should be just a hint of a bite in a kiss—very brief, just a playful glimpse of what could be.

*O*NCE THERE WAS A MAN WHO NEVER ejaculated. He achieved this skill after many months of practice—years, really. He could last so long, women would beg him to stop. And very graciously, he would. He loved bringing his women to the point where they would *plead* with him to stop. He defeated all of them.

The only trouble is he enjoyed his triumph far more than he enjoyed the sex. But he wasn't able to understand the difference. Though in a purely technical sense he was a great lover, he didn't know what he was missing.

A MAN WENT TO A DOCTOR. THE DOC- tor examined him and said, "You'll have to reduce your sex life by 50%." The man said, "Doctor, which 50%? Talking about it or thinking about it?"

People are always thinking about sex. They think about it before, after, during, and instead of. But thinking about sex won't do anything for you. It will only get you agitated. You see, whereas your body is natural, your mind is unnatural. Your body can get enough; your mind can't. If you're caught up in the frantic merry-go-round of constantly and obsessively thinking about sex, you will never feel satisfied. Then therapy is needed, or perhaps meditation, or maybe even such a prodigious overabundance of sex that once and for all in your life you'll feel you've had more than enough.

*H*OW DO YOU EXPERIENCE LIFE? As choice or as obligation?

If you experience life as obligation rather than choice, resentment is inevitable. That's why many people are so full of indignation. And though normally the hurt, angry feelings are unspoken, they're there right beneath the surface. All that keeps the rage from boiling over is hope—hope for some sort of reward if one behaves.

When that hope is gone, people do terrible things. Only two factors keep that kind of violence from erupting: the continuing hope for future rewards (on earth or in heaven) and the deep understanding that it's *your* life, that you can do with it what you want—*that you have choices.*

*T*HEY SAY THAT SEX CAN BE AS GOOD after 65 as at 18. Those who know claim it's often even better—more mellow and less driven, even though there isn't as much jumping around. One man of 75 offers, "I'm still going strong, and I've been interested in sex since I was five! I'm not good-looking, I'm not rich, I may be totally crazy, but I enjoy the ladies and they sure do seem to enjoy me. I'm still a sexual being, and I don't want anyone to forget it!"

But there's always another opinion. A lady of 78 told me, "One disappointing thing about sex is that when you finally get comfortable with it, you're too old to really enjoy it. I mean, you can still enjoy it, but it does start looking a little childish." All depends on who you're talking to.

*I*T'S HARD FOR US TO TAKE RESPONSI-
bility for our own desires. We won't admit
to what we really want. That's why we so often
do—or pretend to do—what others want us to
do. Every kid knows how to make it look as
though he's trying oh so hard to do what Mommy
and Daddy want—so it's not his fault if it doesn't
work, is it?

That's how little devils come into being. "I
did exactly what you wanted me to do" is a
wonderfully effective way of sabotaging others.
We grow up saboteurs, and we carry that with us
into adult life. You can see a lot of this in sex.

Are you aware of your little devil?

O NCE THERE WAS A WOMAN WHO WAS very good at pleasing men. She knew all the tricks, and she rather enjoyed driving men wild. But she herself never felt anything.

One day she met a man who didn't want her to satisfy him. Instead, he looked into her eyes. They spent hours just touching each other in a caring way that was *almost* sexual but not quite. Whenever she tried to satisfy him as she had always satisfied other men, he said, "This isn't about sex. This is about being together." And that's how their lovemaking continued—if in fact you could even call it that.

And then a strange thing happened. For the first time in her life she began to feel—when they finally did have sex—that the sun rose at midnight and they traveled together to the craters of the moon. It was something of tremendous depth and sweetness and of *exquisite* beauty.

They didn't make love again for months. They both knew that the experience had been perfect.

*F*OR MANY PEOPLE—OUR MOTHERS and aunts, perhaps—sex is still a very embarrassing subject. If they have to talk about it, they find it almost impossible to use explicit language. They say the cat "got married" and they avoid words like *coitus, copulate, mate, or intercourse.* When other people use those words, they squirm. This puts them at a disadvantage because one can so easily humiliate them. They are very vulnerable. Use a basic four-letter word in their presence and they cringe. And yet, because we don't want to hurt them, in a way they are very powerful. Silently, with merely a pursing of their lips, a glance, or a tiny grimace of displeasure, they impose their own restraints on our exuberance. They inhibit the way the rest of us talk. They take the joy out of us. That's why we usually visit only for a day or two and leave as soon as we can.

S EXUAL FANTASIES AND DREAMS EN-
rich life. They tell you things about yourself. Why scoff at them? Kinky or not, weird or
not, look at them as you do a movie, and avoid
judgment and revulsion. *Whatever* your fantasy
may be, it is a gift from existence. Above all, try
not to withhold anything from your beloved
that is in your mind.

A sage once advised, "Share not only your
body, but share your mind as well."

I would say: don't shut your lover out. Let
him or her know your fantasies.

*S*EX IS A CHASE AFTER THE MISSING link—the missing link in oneself. The other is seen as the absent segment needed to redeem the puzzle. Though misguided, this approach is at least honest compared to people who pretend they don't crave love, need no one, never have erotic dreams, and "can't understand" what all the fuss is about.

But sex can't really make you feel complete. Nor can another person. Even the best relationship cannot make you feel whole. It isn't that they're not important—sex, love, and relationships *are* important. But something more is needed: a deep connection with self. Lovers, children, friends, and rewarding careers can enrich life, but only if you're already committed to your self—to your core, your soul. Coming back to your self is the only way to attain wholeness. You can't do it through sex.

*S*HAME CAUSES US TO HIDE. WE FEEL AS though we have been stupid or done something revolting—failed in some unfathomable way. What you considered private was publicly ridiculed. And the memory of how we were exposed still haunts us, still makes us squirm, even though it was years ago. You masturbated, or you liked someone, and when that was discovered, you were ridiculed for it. Somebody mocked you by chanting, "She *li*-ikes *Way*-ayne," or "Randy has a *girrrl*-friend!" Maybe you used a wrong word and everyone snickered and guffawed. Maybe you said something that indicated you weren't quite clear about how babies are born, and someone sneered, "Don't you even know *that?!*" So many putdowns! Maybe you went, all eager, to show Dad a pretty picture you had drawn, and he, from behind his newspaper, barked, "Can't you see I'm *busy?*" You cringed and your stomach dropped and you felt like disappearing under the rug. Maybe you're still under that rug to this very day!

*T*HE MIND DOES STRANGE THINGS with sex.

If you make love to someone who isn't sensitive to your needs, the mind concludes, "I never get what I want."

If you make love to someone who *is* sensitive, the mind concludes, "I always get the wimps."

If your lover says he loves what you did, your mind says, "He doesn't love me for me but only for what I do."

If you make love and he satisfies you completely, the mind concludes, "This won't last."

Your mind is so bizarre, it will not only derail your enjoyment, it will even convince you that your enjoyment wasn't enjoyable!

*P*EOPLE HATE WHATEVER HAS POWER over them. That is why some men brutalize women. They think of the woman as synonymous with the sexual organ that has such a powerful hold on them. She is "a cunt." They despise what they feel dominated by. Instead of hating their own hormones, they hate the organ of the woman—and she often hates theirs. We can feel like puppets whose strings are being pulled, and in our confusion think that what's pulling our strings is the other sex.

All that is delusion. What's really pulling our strings is the fear of being overwhelmed with pleasure. We're constantly running after enjoyment and yet we're constantly recoiling from it. Many people give in to their biology only when they absolutely have to, and even then in a very grudging way. We crave secret pleasures, but openly acknowledged and *shared* pleasure is still scary for many.

*T*HE VERY TERM, *OPPOSITE SEX,* IS significant. Why bother saying "opposite" when "other sex" is adequate? You say "the opposite direction" when you can go in any direction. But opposite sex? If you have two children, you don't say "my opposite child," do you? So the use of opposite sex is significant. It is a distancing. It indicates the presence of an emotional charge. It says:

"*Get away!* You have too much power over me and I'm not sure I can handle it."

*D*ON WAS A MILITARY MAN WHO HATED women. But he didn't know he hated women. He only knew he hated his ex-wife. Years after they divorced, Don continued to blame her for everything. Then one day he went to a certain part of the world where he could have sex with lots of different women, as much as he wanted. These were warm, affectionate, loving women, not prostitutes. He wasn't paying them or forcing them, and they were not obliged to be with him. He simply asked them and they almost always said yes.

Overnight, Don went from being deprived and frustrated all his life to having this incredible overabundance for a year or so. And his whole attitude toward women changed. He began to like women! The last I heard he had called up his ex-wife and they'd even become friends. Slowly he saw that it hadn't been her all along—it had been his own rage about being starved for so long. And for the very first time ever, Don was at peace with himself.

S IT BACK TO BACK WITH SOMEONE. Feeling the other person's warmth and holding hands perhaps, allow your jaw and your breathing to relax. Then softly say the words, "I *love* doing this." You should feel as though you are announcing this to the whole world. After a while, sit face to face, first looking and then embracing, and continue reiterating, "I love doing this." Begin gently caressing each other's hands and feet, and as you do, say "I love your doing this." Your partner will then confirm this by saying, "You love my doing this." When it seems appropriate, switch to "I am moving into ecstasy and I love it," with your partner affirming, "You are moving into ecstasy and you love it."

Continue to do very slowly, alternating back and forth. Do it long enough and slowly enough to enter the kind of altered state in which you are supremely relaxed and peaceful.

*F*REQUENCY OF SEX MAY MAKE YOU feel needed. And chances are it will also make you feel good. But it will not necessarily make you feel good about *yourself.* And feeling good about yourself is worth far more than just feeling good. If you feel good about yourself, you feel good even when you feel awful.

Once you feel good about yourself, even the most horrendous tragedies will not destroy you. When you feel good about yourself, you'll still have the same feelings as everyone else—fear, anger, hurt, and so on—but because you know you are basically a wonderful person, such negative feelings will not affect you quite so much.

How can you feel good about yourself? It only requires one thing: genuinely deciding to do so. On these inner planes, you see, everything is sheer magic. When you decide to feel good about yourself, you are beyond mere cause and effect.

*L*IZ BECAME AWARE THAT ROGER OF-
ten started a fight just before they were
supposed to have sex. After a while it dawned on
her that this was Roger's way of avoiding. The
issues they fought about weren't so important;
the *effect* of the fight was to move them away
from sex.

When Liz finally twigged, she said, "Roger,
I've got it! You pick fights just to avoid sex!
Roger, I think you must be *afraid* of sex!" This of
course led to a humongous fight. Once the fight
was over however, Roger admitted he was, in a
way, afraid of sex—he hated the fact that she
always seemed so thoroughly to enjoy it while
he didn't. "Well if *that's* what it is," exclaimed
Liz, "I will teach *you* to enjoy it!" In a sense she
started doing sex therapy with her own mate.
They got so involved in their therapy, the money
they saved by staying home paid for their next
vacation.

*W*OMEN COME TO COUNSELING TELL-
ing me how unhappy they are. Then
they add, "But I don't have any right to be unhappy! Many of my friends complain that their
husbands aren't interested, but my husband is
always interested—he wants to have sex with
me four times a day and seven times on Sunday."

How do I handle that one? Here's this very
nice woman, apparently enjoying a great sex
life, and she keeps asking herself (and me) why
she's so unhappy despite all this incredible lovemaking. So I make like Solomon and this is what
I say:

Frequency of sex will not make anyone
happy. Great sex does *not* guarantee a good
relationship. And even the greatest sex will not
save a bad relationship. The reverse is also true:
bad sex will not destroy a good relationship. No
matter how you look at it, the tail simply cannot
wag the dog.

*S*EX DOES NOT REQUIRE LOVE, BUT IT does require affection and a forgiving attitude. If a person is holding a grudge, it is very difficult to enjoy sex. Sometimes, unfortunately, we have experienced so much hurt that we are unforgiving without being aware of it.

Being unforgiving makes you distrustful. And being distrustful results in having no friends to talk to. So this process of preserving an open wound—which is what not forgiving is—keeps you closed to the possibilities of salvation. It keeps people away from you and it keeps you lonely. Then the only sex life you can have is either with yourself, with someone you tell yourself lies about, or with hired assassins. (I call the people who sell sex "assassins" for only one reason: because going with them tends to assassinate your self-respect.)

I RIS SEEMED TO HAVE IT ALL; SHE HAD three lovely children, a house in the suburbs, and a doctor husband who was very successful. But there was no sex. She and Steve agreed on many things, but somehow they just couldn't seem to revive their sex life. Night after night they yearned for a warm embrace.

One day Steve had sex with a hooker. And though Iris knew nothing about this, she fell in love with Ian, a young carpenter from Wales. Ian was poor and lived in a rented room, but at least he was *interested*. Since Ian had no money, the only places they could go was the park and his room. They had sex all night and Iris was finally in heaven. Steve pretended he didn't mind, which enraged Iris because she knew it was a lie. To her great surprise, she could suddenly see things very clearly. When you are true to yourself and go with your energy, what was previously obscure becomes luminous.

*W*HAT KIND OF SEXUAL ECONOMY DO you live in? Do you live in an economy of scarcity or one of abundance?

If you live in an economy of abundance, you know that shops are full to overflowing and that your credit is excellent. If you live in an economy of scarcity, you worry about getting fired, a depression is just around the corner, the inflation may wipe you out, and there's never enough to go around.

If you feel that many beautiful lovers are coming your way, you live in an economy of abundance. If you feel that getting *this* one into bed was a major achievement, a once-in-a-lifetime bookkeeping error made by an invisible accountant who basically doesn't like you or that getting *that* one to say yes will be an incredible windfall, then you live in an economy of scarcity. My point is that which sexual economy you live in is a projection, a fantasy product of your imagination. Unfortunately, the fact that you believe it will have a decisive effect on any relationship you enter into.

*T*O HAVE SEX, MANY WOMEN MUST first be in love. All too often, they close their eyes and persuade themselves they are in a loving relationship when they're not. They are swept away by a mirage.

After a few experiences of this kind, many women come to the conclusion that all men are pigs.

A cynic would say it was their eagerness for *sex* that made them close their eyes. An idealist would say it was their eagerness for *love*. But the result is the same: a broken heart and the firm conviction that men are swine.

Until such women can accept that sex and love do not have to go together, they will continue to close their eyes. And if they close their eyes, they will continue to be bitter about men.

*H*AVE YOU EVER HEARD OF ANYONE feeding a shark? No one ever did, you know. No one ever feeds a vulture. But everyone feeds puppies. Everybody loves babies. Everyone cuddles kittens. Maybe all that sharks really want is to be treated like puppies, but they sure go about it in strange ways.

One thing is certain: so long as you're a shark, you don't ever have to worry about anyone treating you like a puppy.

O VEREATING IS A NATIONWIDE PROB-
lem. Billions of dollars are spent every
year to help people lose weight. What is never
mentioned in any of this are two tremendously
important sexual reasons for overeating. Many
people overeat because they've given up on
sex—they've resigned themselves to never having a good sex life. Instead, they settle for vicari-
ous sex by reading magazines or watching the
sexy soaps on TV.

Other people overeat for exactly the opposite reason: they have a deep fear that being
slender would make them too desirable. Everyone will be after them, and they won't be able to
cope. This kind of fantasy suggests that they feel
threatened by sex; perhaps they even regard it as
something sinful. When society finally adopts
healthier attitudes toward sex, we won't see so
many people suffering from obesity.

*T*HE BEST SEX COMES FROM LETTING GO of fixed goals, fixed ideas, tensions, fears, opinions, and judgments, as well as the habit of analyzing, of explaining everything, of making excuses, and of thinking you know best.

How do you let go? You just let go! It's like releasing the air from your lungs. But many people don't want to do it because they're afraid of appearing too ridiculously insignificant.

When you let go, you are in a state of awareness of the moment—you aren't far away in your thoughts, you're not anticipating this or that, you're not lost in some abstraction, you're right here in the now, fully alert, and present. Which feels great in and of itself. Then you can smell the coffee and the roses. It's in that "Ah, this!" moment, with all your mental gibberish out of the way, that you're fully primed for some fantastic sex.

*Y*OU CAN LEARN A LOT FROM MASTUR-bating. You can learn a lot about yourself and the areas of your body that give you pleasure. But you won't learn much if you're down on yourself for doing it. If you abuse yourself for abusing yourself, you're in trouble. Actually, masturbating is not abusing yourself; it is delighting in yourself. Abusing yourself is giving yourself a hard time, whether it has anything to do with sex or not.

*T*HERE ARE WOMEN WHO ARE OBSESSED with the idea of doing certain things to certain parts of a man's body. There are men who are obsessed with the idea of doing certain things to certain parts of a woman's body. It's like an invisible cloud that hovers above their heads wherever they go. And all of these responsible, hardworking, intelligent people are usually very surprised that doing these things to another person's body doesn't lead to joy! They can't seem to understand that that's not the way joy happens.

Joy surges in you when you no longer see problems as problems but as opportunities. Joy is a recognition, the recognition of life abundant. What's glorious about good sex is bathing yourself in that rapture, feeling nirvana deep in the tissues of your body. Nobody has to do anything to you.

T HERE'S LOTS OF SEXUAL ENERGY BE-
tween us! But he takes me to a place I
don't ever want to go. He just wants to get off
and I want it to go on and on for hours. I'm lying
there feeling I'm a virgin Indian princess and the
lights are low and the drums are beating, and
then I'm caught by a wave like a surfboard—
carried by a series of waves I can't control, and
the waves lift me to a river in paradise that I
could listen to forever. And then *this* idiot talks
to me about hookers and red garter belts and
strobe lights, and then he says, "*Did you?*" I'm in
heaven, and he's so unaware, he wants to do a
number on my clit."

This story has been told to me by dozens of
women. It's a reminder that you need to get the
dirty pictures out of your head and be in awareness—not awareness of anything but simply in
awareness, because awareness, alertness, being
fully present to the constantly life-giving now is
such an incredible kick in itself.

*S*EX IS A REFUGE FROM ALL THE CON-
stant jabber. Sex and tennis. Everywhere
else you go nowadays there is talk, talk, talk--
radio, TV, meetings. It used to be you could call
someone up, and if they weren't home, that was
that; now you have to lie to their answering
machine. So it's no wonder that people like sex.
It fills a need.

Tennis, of course, has a few advantages; you
can keep your clothes on, stay reasonably clean,
and you don't have to make a total ass of yourself. What's more, you can really whack somebody around in tennis, let them know what's
what and get angry, which you can't so easily do
in sex. Also, tennis has an edge in that you don't
always have to pretend to be so darn loving. But
when you can't find someone for tennis, sex will
do. Or jogging. At least you don't have to listen
to anyone for a while.

*I*T TAKES PRACTICE AND PATIENCE FOR some women to orgasm. It takes a certain amount of know-how. It requires experimenting. But many women feel that their husbands are in too much of a hurry; some were married five or six years before they ever had an orgasm. All that time they took pride in being good in bed and able to satisfy their husbands. But they themselves never had a release.

Many wives bought the old chauvinist idea that a woman's primary purpose in life is to be a dutiful servant. That's one part of the problem—they had too much invested in being good wives. But the other part is that they were genuinely willing to sacrifice their own happiness for the happiness of their loved one. Often that gave them tremendous joy, but other times it brought them resentment. It's a very fine line, and only you can know which side of the line you're on!

*L*ESS DESIRE, MORE FEELING" IS WHAT distinguishes marriage from an affair. Feelings deepen in marriage—provided, of course, that it's a good marriage. And sexual frequency declines. Before you got married, you did it whenever you saw each other; now that you're together so much, you can't always be at it, especially after the first year or so when kids arrive.

But if feelings *don't* deepen, the old itch will still be there; and if the old itch is still there, feelings won't deepen. Whether the chicken or the egg comes first, the spouse who doesn't feel deeply will develop a roving eye for new and more frothy sex partners—especially if he or she didn't deal with that aspect earlier. When you don't sow your oats when it's time to sow them, that itch remains, and it doesn't take much to scratch it—unless, of course, you are able to open very deeply to your feelings.

F AKING AN ORGASM IS THE ULTIMATE deceit, even though practically everyone does it. It creates an inner separation between you and your beloved. But the real point is that by focusing on your partner's feelings, you lose contact with your own feelings. Faking orgasms can make it next to impossible to have any. You may not be hurting your lover, but you're definitely hurting yourself. And faking orgasms is like any other bad habit; it's easy to get into and very hard to get out of.

Pretending you're having an orgasm does get you off the hook. And it may make your paramour feel better. But when you pretend to feel something you don't feel, you can't really pay much attention to what you do feel. It's as though if you fake it, you can't make it. Invest the energy spent on pretending in surveying your own feelings, and who knows what may occur?

*H*ORMONES SURE HAVE A HARD LIFE. They tend to get blamed for what usually has a lot more to do with fantasies. A young man named Christopher made an electrifying discovery on a deserted beach one day. He became aware that every time he thought of his girlfriend—*boom*—he got an erection!

Chris had a scientific mind, so this puzzled him. "Could it be my hormones?" he wondered. "But my hormones are the same *before* I think of Kathy as *when* I think of her. So if it's not my hormones, and she's not here, what is it?" Then he realized, "It must be my thoughts! My own thoughts must be giving me an erection!"

When this revelation came to him, Christopher felt delirious with excitement. He knew, without any shadow of a doubt, that he had grasped the immense power of the human mind. He felt—well, almost exactly the way his famous namesake must have felt when he first "discovered" America.

S OME PEOPLE ARE SCANDALIZED IF YOU masturbate. Other people are scandalized if you *don't* masturbate. The moral of this story is: You may not be able to please everybody, but you can sure please yourself!

Masturbating will make you more interested in sex. It will keep the home fires burning when your loved one is far away. Not masturbating may make you lose the urge, the relish, the predilection, and even the memory.

*O*H YESOH YESOH *YES!"*
Isn't it amazing how positive even people who complain a lot can get at times?

Sex makes people unbelievably positive—good sex, anyway. Beneath our patina of gossipy sophistication, there's an inner child core of wide-eyed enthusiasm just waiting to be released. You can be bored, blasé, cool, aloof, but when your tautness liquefies, when your brittleness melts and your juices percolate your entire being, when someone catapults you up up up and over the brink, the only thing that's left of you is an adoring *"Ohhhhhh...!!!"*

*I*F YOU DON'T WANT THE KIDS TO bother you while you're making love, say so. Hang a sign on your bedroom door that declares "We need to be alone now," or "Doing our business," or something like that. And lock the door, firmly. They'll get the idea after a while. You needn't worry, either, about what your kids are going to think. They'll think: Mom and Dad are doing their thing. They'll get used to it after a while. They'll probably laugh about it, too, because to a child, sex is silly. And that's how it should be. You are in a way being silly, and you might as well acknowledge it. Sex is the most ludicrous thing imaginable. Nothing wrong with being silly, is there? It's usually the only thing that's any fun.

And if you can't laugh about it all, chances are your current sack time is far from the greatest. My fervent hope for you is that locking the bedroom door and not worrying about the kids for a while will help.

*M*ANY MEN WANT TO GET IN SO BAD it drives them crazy, but the average woman doesn't put quite as high a premium on coitus. Women love having a man inside, but they dislike the uncertainty of being left short. The consensus is that intercourse is simply not enough for most women.

Why? It doesn't depend only on a man's ability; it's also a question of physiology. The vagina just isn't as sensitive as the penis—if it were, it would be easy for women to experience orgasm during intercourse, and it's not. The equivalent of the penis is the clitoris, not the vagina, and that fact has *enormous* implications for lovemaking. I mean, if your big toe were the most pleasure-prone part of your body, you'd use that, wouldn't you? Having comparatively little fun *and* risking pregnancy plus all the rest— you'd have to be a masochist, wouldn't you?

*H*ERE'S AN EXERCISE TO INCREASE YOUR energy and release pent-up feelings:

Lie down and make an *ooooooohh!* sound. Bay the way a wolf does at the moon: pucker your lips and go *ooooooohhh!!* Allow your body to go into whatever contortions it wants while you continue baying *ooooooohhhhh!!* Let yourself writhe and wriggle and make grimaces if that feels right. The sound itself will guide you, provided you go into it with full intensity. Put whatever you have ever felt into this—really let yourself go! If the sound wants to change into an *aaaahhh* or an *ohhhhh* or a laugh or a scream or a jumble of irrational words, let it. *Be sure to stop completely at a pre-set time!* This can be anywhere from ten to forty minutes after you begin. Then lie quietly just watching whatever occurs inside you.

I ONCE HAD A CLIENT WHO WAS OB-
sessed with sex. He was always frantic-
ally running after women and continually getting turned down. He was the most hard-up
human being I have ever known.

One day I said to him, "Stanley, I have an
experiment that may work—want to try it?" He
said, "I'll try anything!" I said, "Will you agree to
be celibate for three weeks regardless of what
happens?" He of course thought I was insane,
but after arguing for an hour he said, "Okay, I'll
do it." And do you know what happened? He
suddenly saw women as human beings and not
just sexual objects. He was able to relate to
women in a reasonably nonmanipulative way
for the very first time. He slowed down. He
relaxed. And since he wasn't constantly behav-
ing in his old pushy way, women didn't auto-
matically turn away from him anymore. He
learned a lot from those three weeks. And then
one day a very nice girl came along, and Stanley-
was totally surprised when she actually said yes.

*M*OST WOMEN DO NOT HAVE AN orgasm during intercourse alone. They require clitoral stimulation. That's why some women use vibrators. It's an easy way to achieve orgasm, and you can then relax when you have sex with a man. You're no longer dependent on him and whether he's got what it takes.

Of course, the idea of using a vibrator may be repulsive to you. It is to many. But if you're starved for satisfaction, it will help. Remember, a vibrator is not intended to replace a man. In fact, it allows you to be with a man in a more relaxed way.

But vibrators can dull your sensitivity. They facilitate one quick fix, but they curtail your receptivity to the entire sensory spectrum. They can get you hooked on a powerful, satisfying, but very limited experience. They tend to close you to the deepest human interaction. So if you use a vibrator, be careful that it enhances your lovemaking and doesn't ruin it.

A PRETTY NINETEEN-YEAR-OLD SHOCKED everyone by marrying a man of 78. They honeymooned in Hawaii, and when they came back, her friends wanted to know how it was.

"Oh, it was great," she said, "I loved it. We had a *wonderful* time! We made love nearly every night."

"Nearly every *night?* But how is that possible? At his age . . . " "Oh, but he's so young in spirit! We nearly made love on Monday, almost did it on Tuesday, got very close on Wednesday, and practically succeeded on Saturday. We made love nearly every night!"

No wife wants to admit her husband isn't a good lover. The tendency is to fan your vanity by pretending that your mate is second to none in the bedroom. So don't believe everything you hear. The truth often doesn't come out until they've written each other off and have their last fling . . . in the divorce court.

*G*OOD SEDUCERS SOMETIMES HAVE THE worst self-esteem. They suspect there's a flaw in what they're doing—a flaw in *them*. They know that being a good seducer doesn't make you beautiful, doesn't make you lovable, and doesn't necessarily mean you're good in bed. Even though it confers a certain cachet of prestige. Whether you're a Jezebel or a Don Juan, you may just be driven.

Of course, being able to seduce is a definite talent, and one that most people envy. In some respects it certainly pays off, but whether it pays off in the way you want it to pay off is another matter. It may not make you feel better about yourself. In the final analysis, being able to seduce really only means that you are skilled at seduction. That's something you may want to keep in mind the next time someone turns on the charm and tries to seduce *you*.

T O THINK THAT ANYTHING INVOLVING the sex organs is sex is to confuse an instrument with an interaction. You wouldn't think burning skis in the fireplace had anything to do with skiing, would you? You wouldn't think smashing a tennis racquet in rage had anything to do with tennis, or that driving your car over a cliff had something to do with motoring. Yet many people believe that anything that employs the sex organs is sex, and this false belief leads to rape, sexual violence, and other perversions. Too many people make a fetish of the sex organs. Though this is foolish, it's really not surprising when you consider how long candid talk about sex has been taboo in this society. When clothes are no longer designed to tantalize, when nudity is fully permitted, when people are friendlier and more honest, sexual violence will disappear.

*S*EX IS *NOT* ALWAYS GOOD FOR YOU. It isn't good for you if you're sick, or if you're trying to figure something out, or if you're grieving about a lost love, or if you'd rather be with your kids, or if you're painting a picture or trying to write a business plan, or if you don't want to stop being angry. And it's especially not good for you if you just plain simply don't want it. Reason and logic don't have any say in sex; whimsy does. There's a great deal to be said for insisting on your God-given right to occasionally behave unreasonably and even irrationally, so don't ever yield to sex just because someone says you should. Hang in there, and use the situation for improving your ability to say no.

*H*ERE IS A MEDITATION THAT WILL make you feel more loving toward your body. Many women (and men too) hated their bodies until they did this meditation. To do it, you need a warm quiet room and a large mirror. Soft music and candlelight will help.

Undress and sit comfortably in front of the mirror. Gaze at your naked body—you should be able to see all of it. Slowly, methodically, inspect your body and keep looking! Look even where you don't want to look. Continue doing this until you feel more comfortable about looking at yourself. Repeat this meditation several times in the next few days.

Gradually, as my clients studied their image, they started to feel more accepting of their body. They saw beyond their wrinkles and bulges. They saw their soul. Their self image changed, and they were then able to be with their lover with greater confidence. They were able to bring a more secure sense of self to their lovemaking.

*F*ORGET ALL ABOUT "WILL YOU LOVE ME forever?" Don't even think it—it makes everything very weird. It's like a policeman asking, "Are you going to commit a crime?" Makes you cringe. Love is like the oceandeep and vast, but it does have tides. Forever is made up of thousands of happy todays. You can't force anyone to commit, but you *can* set limits on what *you're* willing to do. Make every day joyous and forever will take care of itself.

*T*HE MORE YOU PROLONG LOVEMAKing, the greater your chance of breaking through to new highs. Here's something to try when you have ample time; there may be a surprise in store for you after the first hour.

Make love in any way you choose that will permit you to persevere. It needn't be intercourse--few lovers can last that long—and can even be pleasing yourself. Stay with it—go on and on, and on! Immerse yourself totally. If you're relaxed, you'll discover new intensities of pleasure. Men need to be especially careful not to climax too soon, unless of course they have extraordinarily rapid recuperative abilities.

You need to be totally absorbed, so do this only when you are rested and haven't eaten too much. Be sure you create a conducive ambience. Alcohol is not advisable. If you're available, something entirely new may open up for you. Try it; you have nothing to lose except low-level expectations!

*T*HE MADAM OF A VERY PRESTIGIOUS call-girl escort service once observed that those men who called up and said they wanted a girl they could also talk to were almost always satisfied. At the other extreme were the men who called up and specified certain measurements—38-22-36, or something like that. These men, not surprisingly, were very often not satisfied.

The moral of this story is that if you're concerned with numbers, look for numbers, or do it by the numbers, you're simply not moving in the direction of satisfaction.

$\mathcal{A}$ FTER HER FOURTH CHILD WAS BORN, Dolly began to think about sex in a new way. She began to ask questions. She began to wonder why she always had to say yes whenever her husband was in the mood. Dolly had hardly ever enjoyed sex. Married at an early age, she had always assumed that having sex was her duty, part of the marriage contract. But thanks to snippets of conversation she heard here and there, mostly on TV talk shows, she began to suspect that this was not so. One day when George approached her, she blurted out, "I hate having sex with you and I always have!" This wasn't completely true, but she thought it was, and she began to sob. George, of course, was stunned. From that day on he never imposed himself on her again. Ironically, she finally understood she could say no when he started nagging her for sex—before that, he hadn't even asked. One day she finally refused. That's when they started seeing a counselor. After 14 years, Dolly had begun standing up for herself.

*D*ON'T GO STRAIGHT FOR INTER-course. It makes people very uptight. If she says yes, he will feel he owes her something. If she says no, the tension becomes so heavy the relationship may be on its way out. If *she's* the one who's doing the seducing, he may say yes simply because it's expected, but in his heart he may not really want to. So take your time--talk, play, flirt, hug, cuddle, embrace, caress, hold— all that is fine. But if you push for intercourse too soon, you are undermining trust. "Too soon" means pushing for it when it really doesn't feel right yet, when it isn't easy and natural and relaxed. You don't *have* to push; at the right moment it will happen like a ripe apple falling from a tree. Grab at the apple too soon and you'll discover it's sour.

*L*YNNE HATED REJECTION. SHE WOULD do anything to avoid it. So every time a man became serious, she would find herself sabotaging the relationship, intuitively reasoning that if he really got to know how insecure she was, he might reject her. "If somebody liked me, I'd tell him he was worthless. I'd hurt him before he could hurt me."

Once, when Lynne was younger, she was with a sensitive, intelligent man. "But he kept asking me all these embarrassing questions, and I couldn't stand that. That's why I prefer the company of shallow men."

There's a Lynne in all of us. It's scary to let anyone really close, but it's the only chance you have. Yes, you'll probably get hurt, but who cares? There's something inherent in trusting that feels so good, it won't really matter. Check it out for yourself: pick a person you distrust, and now imagine trusting him or her. I'll be very surprised if it doesn't bring a grin to your lips!

*I*S ANYTHING COMPARABLE TO THE euphoria when your partner sheds those concealing garments and this dazzling body stands revealed, newly sculpted? Suddenly you've come home to that precious world of perpetual nakedness. You look, you touch, and so much starts flowing in you, so many vital juices. Everything becomes liquid, everything stirs. Forbidden fragrances, primeval echoes, haunt the sanctuary your bed has become. You soak up ecstasy through the pores of your skin, and soon you enter a zone of forgetfulness where everything dissolves. Afterward, everything feels fresh, clean, bright, and you cry in each other's arms with the sheer joy of it all. And you both know that *this* is life—not the world of meandering chit-chat, paying bills, and all the rest—but this. Each time is a revelation. Even when it's bad, there's still something about it that is unique. And at its best, you feel totally resurrected.

*W*HEN A LOVE AFFAIR ENDS, WE TEND to think the love wasn't real. He or she didn't really love us. Otherwise, wouldn't they have stayed the course? Wouldn't it have lasted? But that's fallacious thinking. Everything that's vital sooner or later dies—that's the very law of life. We may deplore it, but it's an edict that cannot be ignored. Real flowers wilt after five or six days; does that mean they weren't beautiful? Does it mean they didn't glisten in the sun, didn't share their rejuvenating euphoria with all who could see? Only plastic flowers survive forever, but they lack the haunting fragrance of real flowers. So which would you rather have: a radiant, living, breathing flower that one day will die or a plastic flower that you can keep in a jar forever?

*I*T'S WORTH YOUR WHILE, IF YOU WANT great sex, to create a bedroom that's ideally conducive to intimacy. It doesn't need to be expensively furnished, but it should be clean and uncluttered, have pleasing colors, and not be merely utilitarian; it should inspire a sense of beauty. The bed you use for sex ought to have a special, exotic, other-worldly feeling, almost evocative of an altar. There should be an air of reverence. Some people enjoy making love under a canopy, and you may want to construct one. Soft lighting is immensely helpful, and so is quietly pulsating music. When the whole room feels like a retreat from the hustle and bustle of everyday life, won't you relish the thought of spending time there with your beloved?

*A*LL OF US ARE, IN A SENSE, MULTIPLE personalities; nobody is just one person. So when you're drawn to someone, it's good to find out about all the various personalities of your prospective lover. When you're attracted to a lush 25-year-old body, do you realize that you might also have to deal with the temper tantrums of a three-year-old? When you're fascinated by a woman who seems to be oozing sex from every pore, do you know that she furiously chews her fingernails when she's alone? And when you're turned on to that supremely successful executive, do you see the little boy inside who lives in a private hell because he's convinced he can't make it?

Regardless of who you think you're attracted to, sooner or later you're going to have to deal with all your lover's moods and foibles. When you loathe some of your mate's more repugnant sub-personalities at the same time you adore his or her being—that's when love comes into its own.

*T*HE FEAR OF BEING RIDICULED SHUTS people up. One woman never understood what an IUD was, never wanted to reveal her ignorance, and so never opened her mouth. Obviously—she didn't want to make a fool of herself. Another woman kept forgetting how to insert a diaphragm. Unfortunately, we often pay a price because we don't have the courage to ask such questions.

This kind of inner squelching is our legacy from an educational system that puts competition before cooperation. To avoid the embarrassment of having to reveal what they're really like, people tend to have anonymous sex. It provides the physical warmth that you crave, and it avoids your having to say very much about yourself. Which is quite a lot for someone who's afraid of intimacy. When your concern about making a fool of yourself no longer rules you, your chances of getting the real thing will improve astronomically.

*T*HERE IS SOMETHING ABOUT SEX THAT just naturally makes people laugh. From the viewpoint of those who are not involved, all this fuss about a few inches of flesh is quite hilarious. And if you're too old or too timid to be part of the action, you can still have a good giggle about it. There's many a country where the old crones love to cackle about who's doing what to whom.

Take the story about the spider. You know how lovers will say, "I could devour you?" Well, it seems there's a certain kind of spider—I can't now remember what it's called—which when it mates literally eats its lover. They do this mating dance, and by the time the male comes, he's gone! The female literally devours him. There's no way he's gonna' have a chance to tell the boys about it. As soon as he's done, he's done *for*.

*P*ERSONS WHO ARE AFRAID OF SEX tend to take the initiative. To wait for the other to act is unbearable—the tension becomes too great. "Why wait?" is their motto. Such undue haste then sets the pace for a life long pattern of aggressive sexual conduct that is never overcome. These people I call techies—they know everything about sex from a technical perspective but they usually lack heart. They lack stillness. They can't truly be with another human being. They can't connect.

Techies always take the initiative. That's how you can spot one. They find it difficult to let their partner do things for them. They cannot simply *receive*. They know a lot about sex from a plumbing point of view, but it's all superficial. What good sex requires is receptivity, not elaborate antics. Learning to give and receive gracefully is the key to good sex.

*W*HAT IS SEX LIKE?" THE CHILD wanted to know.

The mother could have said many things. She could have said, "You're too young to ask such questions," or "When you experience it, you'll know," or even "It's great, honey, and one day you'll find out." But she was a wise woman so she didn't.

She just smiled and said, "I like it. You know how you used to feel when I kissed your belly button? And you felt so good you could hardly stand it? That's sort of what it's like!"

D ID YOU EVER HAVE THE EXPERIENCE of thinking you wanted sex and then discovering that you really didn't? Often we're not aware of our deeper needs. We're not tuned in. We're conditioned to think we want sex; sex has become a knee-jerk reflex. But the deeper part of us often wants something quite different—maybe to work in the garden, possibly to sit quietly and pray or meditate, or perhaps to go hiking in the woods.

When we don't listen to ourselves, something goes wrong—some sort of dysfunction. When what you want and what you *think* you want are out of sync, you have to look deep within yourself. Once you learn how to do that, you'll increasingly find what it is you really want at any given moment.

*T*WO WIVES START TALKING. THEY discover they share the identical problem: their husbands are no longer interested in sex. One says, "I'm going to talk to a counselor." The second declares, "I'm going to get a divorce." Just then a third comes along with the same problem and asks, "What's all the fuss about? It's just a question of time until he gets over it."

A major sexual problem to one person is shrugged off by another as a minor nuisance. Your attitude seems to make all the difference between sexual tragedy and sexual farce.

The crucial point is that when a spouse insists on an arbitrary level of sexual performance, the marriage is inherently in trouble. Why? Because with that kind of rigid attitude, it will be just a question of time until performance drops below the requisite level. The very insistence on performance becomes an unbearable pressure. Standing up for yourself in a harsh way may sink your entire ship.

E VERYBODY HATES USING CONDOMS. Whether they're thick or thin, pink or blue, lubricated, ribbed, rolled, with polka dots, or whatever—the plain fact remains that everybody hates using condoms.

Everybody hates using condoms!

Other than that, I can't think of a thing to say about condoms—except that they just might save your life!

Y OUR PELVIS NEEDS TO BE FREE TO swivel and rotate. It needs to be independent of *you*. When it isn't, your enjoyment is curtailed. Most people don't realize this and never know that their sexual feelings are a fraction of what is possible. Once your pelvis is free of you, it begins to move of its own accord. This autonomous movement of the pelvis is the orgasm reflex, and it is not only pleasurable in and of itself, it is a prelude to even greater pleasure.

To free your pelvis, shake your body to pulsating music. Let the shaking begin in the legs and then spread to the rest of your body. Continue as long as it's enjoyable. Then stand with your knees slightly bent, your mouth open, your arms hanging. Rock back on your heels as far as you can without straining. Suddenly you will notice an involuntary quivering beginning. It is this that will slowly free all kinds of blocks in your body.

L ET ME REMIND YOU: SEX ISN'T ABOUT bodies seen from the outside; it's about your body experienced from the inside.

What does that do to voyeurs? It puts a dunce cap on all their collective heads.

The journey to ecstasy is inward. So don't be influenced by the subtle sexual propaganda the slick magazines sell; that's all just deftly veiled pornography and sophisticated teasing. You can just be you. What you experience is what you experience. You don't need to have a perfect body. You don't need to have a perfect anything. Isn't that a relief?

L OVEMAKING IS NOT CONFINED TO the 45 minutes of sex. It does not begin when the lights go out. *Love play begins long before foreplay.* And it is not confined to the bedroom. The way a man and a woman treat each other, the daily acts of kindness, the loving glances, the genuine consideration, the mutual respect—it is this that empowers love. There are couples who make love like this all day and every day, and they may never need to have intercourse; and there are couples who never make love, even when they are engaging in intercourse.

So think of your loved one with affection during the day. Rise to the level where your thoughts are positive. Don't push yourself to think loving thoughts, but rather find the level inside you where thoughts of love and caring already exist.

E XPLAINING THE *FACTS OF LIFE* TO A child isn't easy. Once there was a father who explained the facts of life to his son. At the end, tired from the exertions of having to say what he had never put into words before, he said, "Freddy, now that I've explained it all to you, would you please inform Billy?"

So Freddy went to Billy and said, "Dad wants me to tell you the facts of life."

"Okay," said Billy. "What are they?"

"Well," said Freddy, "you know what we were doing with those girls behind the barn last week? Dad says the birds and the bees do it too." Who is it who really requires an education?

*T*HERE IS SEX THAT MAKES YOU SING, and there is sex that only makes you groan.

Whenever you feel yourself pulled by dark, heavy, murky energy, do this: think of a person, anytime in your life, who has made you feel light and confident. A person who, when you think of him or her, puts spring into your step and brings a happy smile to your lips. If you've never known such an individual, imagine someone like that. Hold that image, focus on it, and it will guide you.

You see, it isn't so much a question of whether you *have* sex or not—it's a question of the *kind* of sex you have. There is nothing wrong with sex as such, it's simply a question of whether it makes you feel lighter or heavier. A song in your heart is worth more than all the hanky-panky, all the pathetic groping with undergarments, and all the little seduction games. It isn't what you do, it's the *spirit* in which you do it.

*T*O A SEX ADDICT, BEING DEPRIVED OF sex is like taking the sap out of the tree of life. It's as devastating as a junkie who is denied his fix. It doesn't matter if the sex has been good, bad, or mediocre; being deprived of it feels like a death sentence. To a sex addict, having sex is synonymous with living, and life without sex is no life at all. So when such a person gets older and has fewer opportunities, the decline of sexual activity is often experienced as a living death, a harbinger of extinction. That's because we don't comprehend that there is a season for sex, a time for the hormones to be racing, and that the later years are designed for a quieter style of life—one in which we can still enjoy sex but whose primary focus is tuning in to the energies of the beyond.

*S*EX CAN BE VERY LOW, VERY ORDINARY. But sex ceases to be ordinary when love comes in. Love transforms sex. It raises sex to a higher level. It purifies sex of all selfishness, all sensual and emotional greed. And once greed is gone from sex, sex becomes something altogether different. A sage once said that sex may be the lowest rung on the ladder of love, but that it's a ladder that can take you all the way to God. When sex is purified, it attunes you to prayer.

*B*EING ATTRACTIVE HAS VERY LITTLE to do with looks. It has to do with attracting, which is what a magnet does. That is a magnet's inherent power. Attractiveness is also a kind of power.

Becoming powerful requires risking. Someone who plays it safe will become neither powerful or magnetic. If you're constantly playing it safe, you won't have real friends—acquaintances yes, friends no. Having friends requires becoming genuine, because that's what real friendship is being genuine with one another. That's the attraction.

Of course, taking risks doesn't, in and of itself, make you powerful. It may only make you a fool. But you can't become magnetic without it. So start to live a little more dangerously—you'll be a lot safer in the long run.

*S*EX INFLAMES THAT PASSIONATE PART of us that we usually keep safely tucked away. Enormous rage suddenly flares up, and we read about it almost daily in the papers.

The crimes committed in the heat of sexual passion have very little to do with sex. The real culprit is our poor lifestyle. If we lived with greater totality, enjoyed life as fully as it could and should be enjoyed, we'd still feel sad when we lost someone, but it wouldn't cripple us. We wouldn't need to take revenge. If you commit to life and live all of life passionately, you won't be so devastated when that special charismatic person says no to you; you'll know that from now on, there will *always* be magical people in your life. And there always will. In fact, with that very realization, you yourself will have become magical!

*M*ASSAGE CAN BE GREAT, BUT NOT everyone likes it; a few people find it irritating. But just try tenderly putting your hand on someone's back and you'll discover it can send electricity up your spine! Of course, you have to let yourself really feel your hand and your partner's back and stay with it. There are other places, too (the top of the head, the butt, the neck, the small of the back, the chest) where softly putting your hand on a certain spot will, after a few minutes, have a fabulous effect. Just touching fingertips is also very sexy, and palm-to-palm contact is quite a turn-on too—provided, of course, that your energy is really in your hands.

*T*HE WORST THING ABOUT SEX IS FEEL-ing used. Especially if you're a woman, because allowing a man in is more than just physical. You're there with your lover and you're saying yes with your eyes and your lips and with every part of you, and your heart is opening more and more and you say Yes, Yes, and every-thing in you is opening more and more and more and you say *Yes Yes Yes!!!* If something then happens to make you feel that you're being used, you feel awful.

There's only one thing that's good about such experiences: they help you realize that you no longer want to put yourself in situations where someone will use you. What's more, having known just how bad being used can make you feel, you will be far more sensitive to how you treat others.

*Y*OU HAVE TO BE ABLE TO TRUST THE other person in order to let go. But can you force yourself to trust? No, you can't—there's no way. So please don't try to convince yourself that you should let go. Trust your distrust—it may be intuition.

*A*DULTS KEEP TRYING TO HIDE THE facts of life from children. But children are clever—they quickly find out the truth.

Little Harvey was assigned to write an English composition on "Where I Come From." So he went to his mother and asked, "Where do I come from?" His mother hemmed and hawed and finally said, "The stork brought you." "And where did Daddy come from?" "The stork brought him too." "And what about Granpa?" "Same thing: the stork brought him."

Harvey wrote all this down. The next day at school he handed in the following composition: "According to my calculations, there hasn't been a natural birth in my family for at least three generations."

A cute story! Unfortunately, every time children are lied to in this way, they lose a little more of their trust in the grown-ups who tell such ridiculous tales.

*M*ANY RELIGIONS SAYS WE SHOULD have sex only to reproduce; we should not have sex for fun. But what they are advocating without realizing it is really animalistic sex, because animals only have sex to reproduce. The human dimension in sex is the dimension of fun: fun is what liberates sex from the tyranny of biology. First fun and then love, but if you take the fun out of sex, love won't be able to raise sex to its highest level. Fun in sex is something uniquely human. Fun is inventive, dazzling, invigorating. And it always involves sharing, whereas animalistic sex is nothing but a mechanical lonely straining, uninspired and monotonously repetitious.

A COUNSELOR WAS GIVING A YOUNG boy a psychological evaluation. "What do you see when you look at this?" he asked. "I see an inkblot." "Yes, but what else do you see?" "I see a couple having sex." "And in this picture?" "I see more people having sex." That's the way the test went; regardless of what the psychologist showed him, the boy always saw sex. As he was leaving he turned to the psychologist and said, "Doctor, do you think I could keep some of those dirty pictures?"

There are people who see sex in everything. They see people touch each other and they immediately think this is sex. They know nothing of human warmth. They can't see the beauty in the human spirit. What will happen to these poor people when they die? You couldn't very well let them into heaven—how could they possibly enjoy it? They wouldn't know what to do with themselves.

B OOZED UP, SAM WAS THE LIFE OF the party. What's more, he unabashedly loved pussy. He was always chasing it, and all his many ladies agreed he was a great lover. There was only one slight problem. Sam couldn't get it up if he didn't have some liquor inside him.

Alcohol helps you numb yourself to sexual experiences that repel you. That's one reason people drink. Wives who are victims of repeated acts of sexual coarseness drink, and the husbands who impose themselves also drink, because they know they are violating their partner and, ultimately, themselves too. Both perpetrator and prey are sickened by what they are doing, but they don't know what to do about it. Enmeshed in addictive and co-dependent patterns, they see no way out. Their fundamental vision of sex, love, and relationship will have to change before they can stop drinking.

*T*EENAGERS ARE HIGHLY SEXUAL. SINCE this is very threatening to adults, what do they do? They control the teenagers as much as they can. And what happens? The teenagers get frustrated and grow up to be frustrated adults—frustrated adults who think about sex all the time!

Parents say they can't allow teenagers to have sex, otherwise they'll run completely wild. But doesn't this indicate how cooped up the parents feel? Anthropologists claim that in tropical cultures such as Samoa and Tahiti, teenagers who were allowed free sex did *not* become delinquent. They didn't just run around, and instead of sassing their parents, they honored them. They sowed their wild oats and grew up quite loving, and now they just laugh about it all. The only ones who don't laugh when they hear this are tight-lipped moralists with vinegar in their veins—the ones who never allowed themselves to have an ounce of fun.

*M*EN WHO THINK THE SIZE OF THEIR penis makes them extremely desirable are like survivors from the ice age. Haven't they learned yet? A large penis is not needed to make a woman happy; in fact, if it's too big, some women will run the other way! So don't take pride if yours is unusually large—unless you're pleased with yourself for being able to terrify the opposition.

*H*OW DOES A WOMAN BECOME A PROS-titute? That's an age-old question. Well, there are two basic ways. They seem different, but they're actually closely linked.

Scenario #1: A girl who feels unloved thinks of sex as no big deal. Guys are always hitting on her, so she's already giving quite a bit away. One day someone gives her money or in some other way teaches her the ropes—how she can make money from what she's already giving away.

Scenario #2: A girl who feels it is wrong to have sex with a man she fancies does so anyway. She soon realizes the man doesn't love her and she feels used. If she believes in chastity, she now thinks of herself as a whore and therefore may eventually become one. Because she thought of chastity as an ideal, she began to think of herself as a prostitute—and whatever it is that you think you are, you become.

*W*HEN YOU CAN'T SAY NO, IT'S OFTEN because you're starved for affection. That's why a lot of people become promiscuous. If your parents weren't affectionate, if they didn't have much use for you, if they were always absent or busy with this or that, you were emotionally deprived. Then the quickest way of covering up your depression is with sex, and you do that just as soon as you reach puberty you suddenly discover that you have a weapon, and sex becomes both your drug and your major form of self-expression. That's the way it works, and the parents who are down on their offspring for being "loose" ought to realize that that is a lot better than being suicidal. And parents, of course, ought to look at how they've contributed to the problem. If you don't take the time to give your children a lot of recognition, you have no right to moralize.

I N ORDER TO COMPENSATE FOR A LACK of sex in their lives, many people over-eat. That's because human beings seem to require at least a minimum of sensations to keep them going, and if it's not sex it has to be food or some kind of thrill—sky-diving, bungee jumping, wind surfing, or espionage. A human being craves spice; in fact, when you eat spicy food, you don't feel inclined to eat quite so much. Basically it's either food, sex, recreation, or a really thrilling career. *How* you get your spice is up to you; but if you don't arrange to get it, you'll bloat yourself with more food than your body can handle.

*T*HERE ARE PEOPLE WHO SAY, "THERE is no more to sex than sneezing." In a way they are right—for them. That is the only kind of sex they have experienced! They don't know anything else. But they would never have said this had they experienced either ecstasy or full orgasm or passion. So when somebody *does* say something like that, there's no point arguing. From now on you'll know what's behind the statement.

*H*AVING SEVERAL LOVERS AT THE SAME time gets you very fragmented. After a while you don't know who you want to be with. When you're with one you're thinking of the other, and when you're with the other—well, it just goes on and on like that. You get so caught up in lying, you no longer know left from right, up from down. When one of your lovers calls up and insists, "But I haven't seen you for a week," how can you say no? After all, you know you don't want any of them to get really mad at you.

How long do you maintain this juggling act? You continue it until you can't stand it anymore. One day the whole thing just falls apart by itself. What happens then? For a while you sleep alone, and though you dread it at first, you quickly discover that you actually enjoy it. The next time you like someone, you decide that this time there's going to be only this one person, no one else—you're not going to get caught up in that ridiculous circus again!

*D*OCTORS DON'T KNOW. ONLY THE exceptional doctor knows more about sex than his or her patients. Until recently, very few medical schools even offered courses on human sexuality. The average doctor has no more than two hours—repeat: two *hours*—of sex education in medical school. Two hours is *nothing!* Yet who does the average person go to with a sexual question? The family doctor! Well, that is *not* the person to talk to. Instead, there are sex therapists and counselors who have had hundreds and even thousands of hours of training. You might have to work up a little more nerve to go see one of them, but I assure you it'll be well worth it.

*A*LL THIS STUFF ABOUT SIMULTANEOUS orgasm is a lot of nonsense. It's a big myth, and a very damaging one. Men and women are so different physiologically that their sexual rhythms are totally at variance. In fact, it's impressive that on some occasions they actually do manage to climax at the same moment. And not only are their cycles different, but they change all the time. To set up simultaneous orgasms as an ideal is absolutely crazy; it's one of those unattainable chimeras that make people feel inadequate.

Have you ever asked yourself *why* it's so important that a man and a woman come simultaneously? What if you *don't* climax at the same time? Will anybody be there with a stopwatch? We run so many races in life that sex ought to be *one* area where we don't race the clock.

*S*EX ALTERS YOUR MOOD. TIMID PEOPLE suddenly become confident. Sheep become lions. Clark Kent becomes Superman. A wallflower becomes a tigress. But what alters your mood even more is taking risks.

Risking gets the adrenalin pumping and you suddenly feel high—it's like an inner hormonal masturbation. When you pick up strangers on street corners, your mood changes from lethargy to extreme excitation. That's why people sometimes run the most incredible risks, ones that make your hair stand on end if you have any—the rush is so great. But if you're getting your kicks in this way, be aware that it has very little to do with sex. You may as well be robbing banks! In fact, persons who get their thrills in this way run far more risks than actual bank robbers—and all for such a preposterous payoff!

P EOPLE WHO ARE CAREFUL WHEN IT comes to casual sex seem to drop all precautions once they're in a relationship. Their reasoning is, "He's nice, so why do I have to take precautions?" It's like when your mother told you not to talk to strangers—"Mom, he's not a stranger, he's nice."

Nice has nothing to do with it—a disease is a disease. It is impersonal. It can kill you even if you get it from the nicest person in the world. The most wonderful lover can quite unintentionally give you the most horrendous disease. It may not be his or her fault—no one's *intentionally* giving it to you, of course—but you're infected nonetheless. Yes, it's annoying to take precautions, but you still need to take precautions—*adequate* precautions—even with the nicest of lovers. If you don't . . . well, read the newspapers.

*D*O YOU KNOW WHY THERE'S SUCH AN unending barrage of dirty jokes? A philosopher once said, "Man suffers so deeply that he had to invent laughter," and sex is an area in which people suffer a great deal.

Sexual wit is very liberating. It is the humor of release. By inducing laughter, it releases tension. Telling an off-color anecdote allows you to express your embarrassment, your anxiety, and your apprehensions indirectly, without having to reveal anything personal. You may disapprove of dirty jokes, but they do enable us to talk about topics we're unable to discuss otherwise. They make it easier for people to confide in each other. They are an escape valve for our concerns. So the next time you hear someone telling a filthy story, have pity—what else is the poor sap supposed to do?

*L*OVE IS LOVE. SEX IS SEX. YOU CAN have sex *with* love, and you can have love *with* sex, but basically, love and sex are different. Of course, there's a lot of resistance to looking at life like that. In practice, it comes to "I love to be with her, therefore I'll have sex with her," or "I want to have sex with him, therefore I know I love him." All this perpetuates an illusion. Love is love. Sex is sex. Both are beautiful, but they are as different as . . . as they are. They merge at a certain point, but you don't get to that point by withholding either one or the other. Or rather, you don't get to that point of melting with an attitude of withholding.

*S*OME PEOPLE SEEM TO KNOW HOW TO do just about everything. They know how to raise children, they know how to keep books and file taxes, they know proper etiquette, they know how to sail, they know how to decorate a house and how to repair the plumbing, and they know how to make people feel at ease. Amazingly, the only thing they don't seem to know how to do is find an outlet for their sexual needs. Poor people! I guess we'll just have to let them go on being perfect until they decide it feels a lot better to be human.

And if you feel you're just a tad like this, please do a little homework; ask yourself why it's so necessary for you to ignore your very basic human needs. What for? And when you've figured that out, kindly do something about it!

*O*NCE THERE WAS A MAN WHO FOUND it very difficult to say what he wanted, no matter who he was with. Instead of being direct about his desires, Mr. Friedman would always say, "In Thailand . . . " Then he'd say what it is they do in Thailand, which included all his favorite fantasies. The truth was he had never been to Thailand. It was a very round-about way of communicating his sexual prefer-ences, but it was the only one he could manage.

*H*AVING A SECRET KEEPS YOU SEPA-rate. The nature of the secret doesn't matter; what matters is that being separate makes you lonely. The loneliness is painful and hard to endure, so it's not surprising that a person turns to sex in order to relieve it. Sex is a balm that fixes the loneliness—momentarily. But as this process speeds up, addiction is born.

To get out of sexual addiction, you first need to get out of loneliness. To get out of loneliness, you need to share your secret with people you can feel safe with. You escape the cycle of addiction in the exact reverse order in which you entered it.

*T*HE VICTORIANS THOUGHT IT EX-
tremely clever to talk about sex without
using any words that overtly related to sex. They
became masters of sexual innuendo. This had a
certain unexpected backlash; it sexualized everything and made everything dirty. Everything
became tainted with double entendre. It's like
the word *gay* in more recent times, you can't
really utilize it anymore for what it used to
mean. Of course, given the censorship laws the
Victorians lived under, they had no choice but to
develop subterfuge. But the whole thing led to a
lot of sneakiness.

That's what happens when you try to out-
law something—sex, drugs, or what have you. It
just comes back at you in some unexpected way.

*T*HERE'S ONE AND ONLY ONE ABSO-
lutely true thing about sex. It is that
when it comes to talking about sex, most people
lie. People who claim they're not interested in
sex lie. And people who *are* interested in sex also
lie.

Those who participate in sex lie in one way
and those who don't lie in another. Non-partici-
pants tell unimaginative and stodgy lies: "I'm
not interested"; "I'm not attracted"; "I find it all
rather revolting," and so on. Participants tend to
tell flattering lies; "Yes, I enjoyed it" is their
biggest. "I'll call you soon" is another. "I just
love *everything* about you" is a humdinger of a
lie. "Oh, that feels so *good!*" is a lie when you're
angry at your lover and feel like poking his eyes
out. "It was great" is probably the most frequent
lie. When we don't focus on honesty, when we
don't strengthen our spine with truth, sex inevitably becomes a lie.

Truth is life-giving, lies are life-annihilating.
And only the truth will set you free.

*M*OST MEN THINK THEY ALWAYS need to be ready to perform. So when a woman touches them, that's what her touch triggers—not the pleasure of that touch but a thought balloon over their head that says "I've got to get it on." Men are so conditioned to perform that a woman's daintiest touch often sets off something like an eight-point earthquake reading on their Richter scale.

Too many men think that if a woman touches them affectionately, they are being asked for sex. It's not so—physical affection is not necessarily a prelude to sex. For many women, touch is at least as desirable.

So men, if every time your woman touches you, your inclination is to relate to it as something sexual, you'll be turning her off, not on. She may not want sex on those occasions, and she may conclude that it's better not to touch you at all if you so often get the wrong idea.

*H*UMAN CURIOSITY IS ENDLESS. LUCKily, it doesn't take us long to realize when we're being overwhelmed with excessive information. When her class was assigned a book report, 13-year-old Amanda decided to read the Masters and Johnson classic, *Human Sexual Response*. "That's not a book someone your age should be reading," her teacher said. "You won't be able to understand it." Amanda, however, was an independent soul, and she insisted she would be able to understand it. By the time the report was due, the teacher was curious what Amanda would say. The book report opened with these words: "I learned more about sex from reading this book than I ever wanted to know ...." She understood instantly how much she missed innocence.

*T*HE OTHER DAY ON A TV TALK SHOW I saw a therapist telling a happily married couple they needed to sleep in the same bed. Their insisting they preferred separate bedrooms was to no avail; she wagged her finger at them and harped, "You are afraid of intimacy!"

This is the kind of thing that gives therapists a bad name. It is meddling and trying to intimidate someone with expertise. Everyone is afraid of intimacy, so you can level that kind of accusation against practically anyone. I think this kind of stuff is frankly quite awful, and I hope you don't pay attention to such junk.

Be very careful of therapists who browbeat you with antics like this. A therapist should *never* take a superior attitude. If one does, that ought to tell you right there that he or she is not a good therapist. Whether or not you sleep in the same bed as your lover is a purely personal preference. So please go ahead and do whatever feels good to you.

*T*HERE ARE MANY WAYS IN WHICH people deal with their fear of sex.

They overeat.

They overwork.

They get sick.

They get obsessively involved in a cause.

They become caretakers.

They suddenly find something very important they have to do, like pay bills or clean the house.

They never go out alone.

They have accidents.

They become destitute.

They have only totally safe relationships.

They won't compromise their ideals.

They refuse to settle for a less than perfect mate.

*O*NCE THERE WAS A WOMAN NAMED Sybil who went around telling her friends how great her sex life was. She had *this* kind of orgasm and that kind of orgasm, and they did it all night for so-and-so many times, and it was all incredible and so on and so forth. And then one day Sybil killed herself.

Her friends thought this was very strange. After all, if your sex life is so great, how come you are killing yourself? But they couldn't ask Sybil that, because she was dead. Obviously, something wasn't right in this great sex life of hers. That's the way a lot of people are—they tell you how great everything is. They can't admit things are not great. So they get very caught up in their own fantasies. They see things a little out of perspective. If Sybil had admitted that her *life* was not quite as great as her legendary *sex* life, maybe something could have been done. But she was too proud for that.

L ITTLE WILLY WAS TOLD THAT IF HE didn't stop masturbating, he would go blind. A week later, what do you think happened? His father discovered little Willy going at it. "Look, Dad," little Willy said in his defense, "it feels so good—couldn't I just go on 'til it's time to get glasses?"

A generation ago, people still thought masturbation could lead to all kinds of terrible things—feeblemindedness, degenerate offspring, and so on. It can't. That is all nonsense. And yet millions of people led tormented lives because they believed this stuff. They were scared stiff, but they just couldn't stop. One woman says she never even knew that other women masturbated; she thought she had to go to bed with a man to get satisfaction, and because of that belief she got into a bad marriage. Nowadays we know that masturbating is normal and not in the least unhealthy. Research even indicates that it is the most common form of sexual satisfaction there is.

*W*IVES COME TO ME AND ASK, "WHAT can I do? My husband doesn't want to change—he doesn't even want to hear about any of this." And I agree that that's a tough situation. I don't know what they can do, and I freely admit it. What, after all, can you do with someone who doesn't want to open his ears?

But then I add that incredible changes are sometimes possible in one spouse if there is a significant change in the other. If a wife lets go of her ideas of how things ought to be, a husband will pick up on that and he'll eventually respond. When he isn't being pulled hither and thither, when a wife neither whines nor pleads, when she frees herself from co-dependency, when he isn't being pressured, something unforeseen can happen in the husband. Sometimes, a result that you ardently desired but couldn't achieve emerges seemingly by itself, except it's even better. That is the magic of letting go. When we let go of our fixed ideas, the whole world changes.

*Y*OU DON'T HAVE TO DISCUSS THE mechanics of sex with your lover ("Put you fingers here, squeeze," and so on) but it *is* a really good idea to be able to talk to your paramour about the quality of your sex life, about what you experience—not nitty-gritty details, but sharing an overall view to convey what the experience means to you.

The meaning of sex is a question that is rarely considered, and yet if sex isn't meaningful, it's really rather perfunctory. So explore the significance of sex by examining its meaning with your partner. Talk with him or her not only about what you feel *in* sex, but also brainstorm how you feel about sex and its relevance to both your lives.

E VERY SEASON HAS ITS OWN DELIGHTS. The intoxicating sex of young love is different from the kind of sex you have later on. The first few months, everything you do sexually is so urgent that it's like a matter of life and death. But later on, when you're not quite so keyed up, your lovemaking will have a different dimension, a different flavor—more relaxed and sweeter. It can bring tears to your eyes and melt your heart. Your knowing this and understanding it is vitally important. If you don't, you'll anticipate at Thanksgiving what was appropriate on the Fourth of July. Mangoes in December might be nice in the supermarket, but when it comes to sex, remind yourself not to expect exotic fruits out of season. If you do, you'll have to start shopping at some other store.

*W*HAT SEX IS REALLY ABOUT IS THE magic of meeting another person. It isn't so much about orgasm or love as it is about magic. It is a sudden unexpected meeting in which one person gives everything—totally—that can be given by one human being to another. It is about nakedness and it is about mystery. It isn't about what you do together, it is about meeting—a meeting that transcends time, worry, and ambition. It is a moment of truth, an unforgettable glimpse of eternity. It is about the transcendence of all the usual parameters through which we relate. The more you try to hold on to your power, influence, and status, the less likely it is that such magic will occur. Letting go of all those safeguards requires courage, of course, but the ultimate gift to yourself and your friend would be to disregard the obstacles and to allow that miracle to transform you.

*W*E *SEEM* TO TALK A LOT ABOUT SEX. But the talk is mostly banter, ribbing, superficial teasing. We skirt the specifics of our own sex life, and we rarely ask our partner significant questions. It's still a delicate subject. For practically everyone, it's still easier to have sex than to talk about it, even with the very person they're having sex with. We avoid asking our dear lover about his or her previous sex life, even if that might protect us from life-threatening infections. Rather bizarre, isn't it?

That it's so hard to talk about sex, to ask about sexually transmitted diseases, is a sign of how much we continue to divide ourselves in two. Though we enjoy sex, we obviously still feel there is something wrong with it. My recommendation is that we reverse that by insisting on open public discussions that view sex as our common personal experience.

*W*HEN YOU GO TO BED WITH SOME-one, you also go to bed with their karma. This may be crystal clear when it comes to something like AIDS or herpes, but it's not so obvious in terms of more subtle psychological stuff. Without getting fancy and esoteric, I'll just say that when you have sex with someone, they get their karmic hooks into you. Intentionally or unintentionally, they manipulate you in terms of their needs, their goals, their dramas, even their sense of propriety. They work on your mind and get you involved in their destiny. Even if you never see them again, they leave an impact. So you want to be very careful who it is you go to bed with. All that glitters is definitely not gold.

*S*EX CAN DEFINITELY BE AN ADDICTION, and it's an addiction with lots of victims. To get out of it (to extricate yourself from any addiction, in fact) you need friends. Friends are not just cronies; friends are people you can really talk to, people who have been there themselves—people who are ready to share their soul without demanding that you do likewise.

Even more than therapy, what we all need today is community, the community of true and responsive friendship. Only the kind of friendship that allows us to talk honestly about our sex lives will liberate us from our nightmares. Only compassionate community will permit us to evolve from the sexual dark age we still live in to an age of friendship, truth, love, and sexual enlightenment. And that, knowingly or unknowingly, is something we all yearn for.

*D*O THE GENIUSES WHO SO COM-
placently tell teenagers to say no to sex
actually believe that even though "say no to
drugs" didn't work, saying no to sex will work?
Teenagers always do what you tell them not to
do, and they've been doing so since grass was
green. Syphilis didn't stop them, pregnancy
didn't stop them, even the threat of castration
never stopped them—sex is simply too powerful a drive. My solution to the AIDS crisis is to
say to them: enjoy sex but do it *intelligently*—and
then to whisper in their ear that tantra is a great
alternative.

Tantra avoids the big explosion in order to
have a more profound experience. In tantra, you
really don't have to "do it." Body fluids don't
have to merge. All you have to do is let your
energies mingle.

Yes, biology is very insistent. But you don't
have to let yourself be stampeded by it. You can
enjoy sex in a different way, as pure energy, until
both of you feel confident you're completely
safe.

S EXUAL DESIRE DISORDERS ARE BUZZ words these days. Behind the jargon is the fact that he wants to when she doesn't, or that she's turned on when he's pooped. And behind *that* is a question of values and priorities. Where do *you* put your emphasis? On financial security or on feeling ecstatic? On being applauded by others or on deepening the closeness between you and your beloved? When you're working all the time, raising children, preparing meals, figuring out your investments, shopping for gifts, doing your taxes, and who knows what else, where's the time for love play?

Add to that the fact that many people feel guilty about sex. Regardless of how much we enjoy it, we don't want to be selfish or "irresponsible," so we put sex on the back burner. Deep down we feel it's really not quite proper. Because of such values, we neglect sex, and so we miss out on its tremendous capability for daily renewal.

*E*VERYBODY KEEPS TALKING ABOUT THE environment. But what about the correlation between sex and the environment? So long as we talk about sex in a cynical, disparaging way, we won't feel the prayerfulness of life. Only when attitudes toward sex change—when it is no longer perceived as something ordinary—will there be real love toward the environment. By celebrating the blessedness of sex, a whole new way of life will be born, and many of our dreams for a new world will finally be fulfilled. And it will happen without violence or bloodshed.

It's up to each one of us to prepare the way. How we express ourselves when we talk about sex can truly make a difference. Our bringing a sense of holiness to life—a merry sense of the sacred, not a solemn one—will be infectious.

*S*EX IS LINKED TO THE DIVINE, BUT IT has become a bargaining chip—an agreement, an arrangement, a tranquilizer. To use it in this way is like milking a cow that is quickly going dry; it is imposing an essentially addictive, workaholic attitude on your deepest stream of life. Without the ecstatic, sex rapidly becomes boring, repetitious, mental. And folks, the ecstatic doesn't happen when all you want to do is fix something.

S OMETIMES IT HAPPENS JUST BEFORE you give up. You haven't connected sexually for weeks, and you've gotten nowhere trying to explain how you feel. You've decided it's useless even *trying* to communicate any longer, and you think that maybe you ought to separate. At that moment, still feeling this pain in your heart, you see her or him, and since you both know words are useless, all you can do is hug.

You hug almost as if you were saying good-bye—and to your utter amazement, there is suddenly so much love in that hug. And—can it really be?—yes: suddenly there is so much sexual stirring! And that stirring, which you could never have imagined, is on a deeper level of sexual love than you ever experienced before. For the first time in a long time there is hope and a kind of knowing. "If we can just keep from arguing," you whisper to one another, "maybe things can work out after all!"

*D*ON'T THINK OF YOUR LOVER AS doing something *to* you. Think of your lover as doing something *with* you.

When someone does something to you, the tendency is to gossip about it. Not only that, but you're not really there. When someone does something with you, it's a shared event, a sacred memento, a little secret you cherish forever that's just between the two of you. It's a very different experience.

What makes the difference is your totality— how much you decide to participate. Once you see that holding back really doesn't do much for you, my guess is you'll decide to jump into it very quickly.

I T'S MY LIFE!" WHEN THIS IS SAID TRULY and not merely in defiance, vistas open up, opportunities arise, creative potential manifests in you to an ever increasing extent. The moment you truly claim your life, you become capable of saying *Yes* and *No*—not before. So becoming powerful is increasingly viewing your life as yours and not someone else's. That's why people who are dying are sometimes so powerful—faced with death they realize it really is their life, *and with that realization they reclaim it.* It's possible at any moment. And once you've reclaimed your life, you can shape it in your own way. So throw your arms to the heavens and forcefully proclaim, *"This is my life!"*

For more about sex as an art, I recommend Margo Anand's *The Art of Sexual Ecstasy*, Paul Pearsall's *Super Marital Sex*, and Dagmar O'Connor's *How to Put the LOVE Back into Making Love*. Charlotte Davis Kasl's *Women, Sex, and Addiction*, Barbara De Angelis' *How to Make Love All the Time*, and Steven Carter and Julia Sokol's *What Really Happens In Bed* are also pertinent.

Osho Rajneesh's books are all fabulous eye-openers, especially *From Sex to Superconsciousness; And The Flowers Showered; The Mustard Seed;* and *Only One Sky*. And I think you'll enjoy the little books I wrote with Judy Ford: *How To Find A Lover, Friend or Companion; Gardening Techniques To Allow Your LOVE To Grow;* and *Lovers' Quarrels*.

Other authors who shaped my thinking include R.D. Laing, Wilhelm Reich, Henry Miller, Alexander Lowen, Rollo May, Ram Dass, Karen Horney, Arthur Janov, Chögyam Trungpa, Virginia Satir, Haim Ginott, Alice Miller, Albert Ellis, Patrick Carnes, and Isaac Bashevis Singer.

WILLIAM ASHOKA ROSS, a therapist for over 20 years, was born on Valentine's Day in Vienna, Austria, became a war refugee at the age of eight, and has been traveling ever since. After college at UCLA, five years as a filmmaker in New York, and a career as a marketing consultant in Italy, he moved to London where he studied with R. D. Laing, Gerda Boyesen, and Caron Kent, and started the Kaleidoscope personal growth center. He led bio-energy and awareness groups all over Europe, lived in Paris, and then went to India to be with Sai Baba and Osho Rajneesh, whose teachings he compiled in *Words From The Masters: A Guide To The God Within*. After many adventures he settled in Seattle to live with Judy Ford, a woman he still finds endlessly inspiring. His "In Your Own Way" seminars are a unique blend of love, therapy, meditation, and miracles. To subscribe to his "Morning Glory Gazette" newsletter, write to him at P.O. Box 834, Kirkland, WA 98083-0834.